A Dairy Tale:

The Ultimate Guide to Pumping, Bottle Feeding and Back-to-Work

Michelle McKeown Poole MS, RN, IBCLC
Illustrations by Elizabeth McKeown, BFA

A Dairy Tale: The Ultimate Guide to Pumping, Bottle Feeding and Back-to-Work

ISBN: 978-1-7345287-1-8

Table of Contents

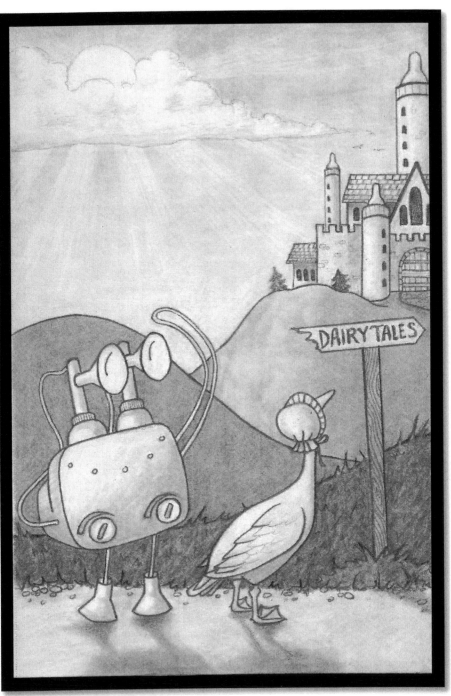

INTRODUCTION

Once upon a time, a beautiful princess gave birth. The royal baby latched without hesitation, and the milk flowed like a torrential river. Pumping came easily to the princess, and the Kingdom's underground ice caves were quickly bursting at the seams with vessels of frozen milk. When it came time to go back to work (she volunteered at the Unicorn Rescue), the princess was able to maintain a mighty milk supply, and stories were told far and wide about how her baby switched effortlessly between bottle and breast. At the appointed time, the princess banished the evil spirit "Mastitis," and gracefully weaned her baby.

And they lived happily ever after.

Fairy tales are great fun, and flood us with happy feelings. As an adult, you might feel removed from these childhood tales…but I think we enter the realms of fantasy daily, whenever we go online. Social media is a place where many parents present their lives as a fairy tale: their grass is always green, their kitchen is always clean, and there is no baby spit-up to be seen. These fictional stories can cause issues for those of us trying to figure out how to feed our babies "the right way," because if we don't know what's real, it's easy to start basing our expectations on a fantasy world—and then feeling bad when our real-life experiences don't measure up.

But never fear! I'm here to break the social media spells, and set you free from the myths, mysteries and mayhem that surround pumping and bottle feeding.

My goal is for you to harness the good feelings and happy outcomes of fairy tales…and use them to create your own version of real-life "dairy tales!" When you're done reading, you'll be a pumping pro.

In this book you'll find ways to:

- Maximize your pumping output.
- Calculate the perfect freezer stash.
- Bottle feed in a way that protects breastfeeding/chestfeeding.
- Feel confident about going back to work.

Before we jump into it, I'd like to quickly cover how your body makes milk, and how to get your supply off to a strong start. (You can find a more detailed review of these topics in my book "Breastfeeding 101: Prepare for the Suck.")

How Your Body Makes Milk

Milk making is based on a supply-and-demand system. A nursing baby or a pump sends the hormonal demand to your brain, "make milk!" and your milk supply increases in response. I.e., the more often you pump or breastfeed/chestfeed, the stronger the "make milk" signal becomes, and the more milk you will make. The less often you pump or breastfeed/chestfeed, the weaker the "make milk" signal becomes, and the less milk you will make. It's a direct relationship, and while you may not always feel like it, you're in control.

Three Ways to Get Your Supply Off to a Strong Start:

1. Before you give birth, learn the basics of lactation by taking a class and/or reading a book.

2. Begin nursing your baby as soon as you can after delivery. Most babies latch within the first hour after birth. If your baby doesn't latch well or

you're choosing to exclusively pump, start pumping within the first few hours, as this seems to help promote a strong milk supply.[1]

3.   Eight good breastfeeding/chestfeeding or pumping sessions every 24 hours is the minimum needed for most parents to call in a full milk supply. "Good" nursing/pumping means it is comfortable for you and effective in getting your baby fed. If you are unable to get in the "magic number" of eight breast stimulations every day, you will still make milk, but not a full supply, and will need to supplement with formula.

Armed with this knowledge, you can combine nursing your baby with pumping and bottle feeding (and/or formula feeding), to create your ideal situation.

Opinion: You Know What's "Best"

I am confident that you know what's best for you, your baby, and your family. Breast is definitely not "best" for everyone, and making parents feel like they're falling short based on how they feed their baby is unfair and unkind. If you are responding to your baby's needs with love and attention, you're doing a great job, whether you're breastfeeding/chestfeeding, formula feeding, and/or pumping and bottle feeding. Your baby thinks *you're* "the best" for meeting their needs in whatever way works.

Language Note: *When talking about babies, I'll use the "they" pronoun to include babies of all genders. And I'll refer to the adults as "mothers," "partners" "parents," and "caregivers." You'll see "breastfeeding/chestfeeding," to include parents who relate more to the word "chest" than "breast," and I'll also use the term "nursing your baby" as a more non-gendered way to talk about lactation. All are welcome here.*

Are you ready? Let's get started!

PART I:
Once Upon a Pump...

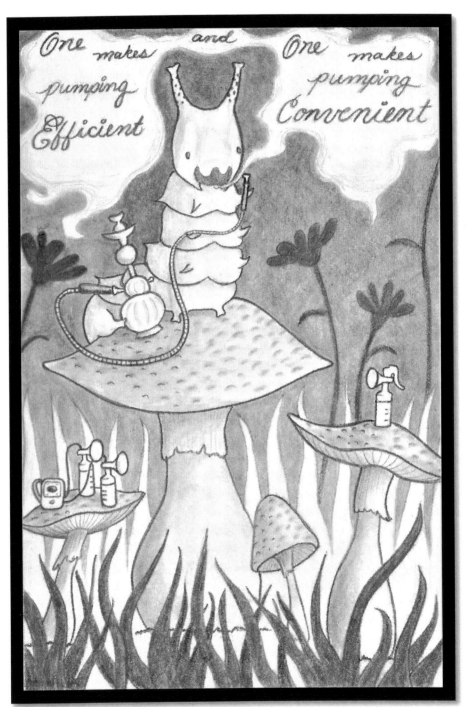

CHAPTER ONE:
WHAT KIND OF PUMP DO I NEED?

There's a lot to think about when it comes to choosing a pump: What kind of pump is best suited to your needs? What are the differences between them? Do you need more than one? By the end of this chapter, you'll know which pump(s) you need, and why.

Pump Options

Double Electric, Single-User Pump. This is the pump you want if you'll be pumping on a regular basis, and the "standard" version (more on this soon) is free through most insurance plans. It is a "double" pump because it allows you to pump both breasts at the same time, which helps you produce more milk more quickly, versus pumping each side separately.[2]

To help you better understand your double-electric pump options, I'm going to break down them down into three categories: "standard," "portable," and "wearable."

A standard pump is the largest of the double-electric pump options and uses tubing to connect the flanges to the pump's motor. Many of these pumps need to be plugged in during use, but there are some with back-up battery options. Standard pumps are free through most insurance plans, whereas most portable and wearable pumps are available only as "upgrades" (which means you have to pay a portion of the price). Although less mobile than the other options, standard pumps are overall extremely efficient and reliable, and therefore a great choice if you are willing and able to sit down to pump.

A portable pump is significantly smaller than a standard pump, but still uses tubing to connect the flanges to the motor, which makes it bulkier than the wearable pumps. These pumps run on a rechargeable battery so that you can move around while pumping. Some provide lanyards and clips to enable "hands-free" pumping, and some don't—so do your research if easy mobility is important to you.

A wearable pump is two small, separate, self-contained pumps, one for each breast. This pump is for parents who are unable to sit down and pump, or who need to be as mobile and discreet as possible.

While the wearable pumps are great, there *are* a few down sides:

- The learning curve is steeper as it's hard to see how the flanges fit and how the controls impact your milk flow...and these factors impact how well the pump will empty your breasts.
- Some wearable pumps don't allow you to switch between stimulation and expression modes.
- The ability to massage and compress your breasts/chest while pumping is limited.

As you'll learn in Chapter Six, the points on this "cons" list come in to play when trying to increase your milk supply, and so you may be at a slight disadvantage if you have a low supply and only a wearable pump to work with. And while these pumps are definitely more discreet than standard pumps, they will still add a few inches (and a little noise) to your bustline.

Single Electric, Single-User Pump. The difference between the double-electric and single-electric pumps is that the single-electric option comes with only one flange. Why would anyone choose this pump over a double-electric?

- It's significantly cheaper if you're paying out of pocket.
- With only one flange, it's more compact.
- You only pump occasionally and so the extra time spent pumping each breast separately isn't a big deal.
- You only ever pump one side at a time.

Please Note: *A "single-user" pump means you shouldn't share or sell your pump, nor should you use a secondhand pump. This is due to the risk of pumped milk becoming contaminated by bacteria and/or mold that are possibly lurking in or on a used pump. Used pumps also might be less efficient, which could cause a mother's milk supply to drop.*

Check if your electric pump is an "open" or "closed" system.
- **In an open system,** there is an opening between the flanges and the tubing. This creates a low risk of milk and/or condensation getting into the tubing. If you own an open-system pump, you'll need to check your tubing for milk and moisture after every pumping session and clean them if you find any, according to the manufacturer's instructions.
- **In a closed system,** the flanges are designed in a way that makes it impossible for milk or condensation to get into the tubing. If you have a closed system, you'll never have to clean your tubing.

Double Electric, Multi-User Pump (aka "Hospital-Grade" Pump). The hospital where you deliver will have a hospital-grade pump on hand, should you need to pump during your stay. This pump is designed to be used multiple times a day, for many years, by thousands of hospital patients. For that reason, it's built with a large industrial strength motor and costs significantly more than a single-user pump.

If you are planning on exclusive pumping or fall into it (e.g., your baby isn't latching), there are benefits to using the hospital's pump while you're there, and possibly renting one upon discharge.

Because the multi-user pumps have a more powerful motor, they tend to produce a stronger suction than a single-user pump. But as you'll read in the next chapter, a higher suction level doesn't necessarily mean more milk. And a good single-user pump provides more than enough power to maintain your milk supply.

Hand or "Manual" Pump. This is a nice pump to have in addition to your double-electric pump. You squeeze and release a manual pump's handle to replicate the pull-tug motion of an electric pump.

- You might use a hand pump when:
    - The power goes out or your pump breaks.
    - You are going out and will need to pump, but don't want the hassle of bringing your electric pump.
    - Your baby starts sleeping longer stretches at night (yay!), and you start waking up in puddles of milk (boo!). This pump makes it easy to take out just a little bit of milk and go back to sleep.

One-Piece Soft Silicone Pump. While the pumps above actively remove milk, this pump collects milk through passive suction.

Many moms think the purpose of this pump is to catch milk that leaks from the opposite breast during feeding. However, it's important to understand that this pump isn't passively "catching" milk—it's actively *pulling* milk. And even though the pull is less than that of an electric pump, it is still breast/chest stimulation, and therefore working to increase your milk supply. While this sounds like a good thing, too much milk, or "oversupply," can easily become problematic (pg. 28).

Therefore, if you're planning on using this pump to "catch" milk, just be mindful of where your milk supply is at and where you'd like it to be, and understand that this pump is having an impact on those things.

Also, know that it's normal to leak from the opposite side your baby is feeding on once your milk supply increases around day three, but this usually stops on its own after the first two weeks, if you just leave it be.

Here are some other ways you might use a silicone pump:

- When you're away from your baby or pump and have milk leaking out of your ears (keep this pump in your bag for emergencies).
- When you're weaning and need to take just a little bit of milk out during the skipped feed/pump to get comfortable.
- When you're looking for an easy way to boost supply (i.e., parents with a low supply actually *want* the extra stimulation this pump provides).

And that's it for pump options!

To summarize: Most pumping parents will want a double electric single-user pump, and a backup manual pump.

Washing and Sterilizing Pump and Bottle Parts

Sterilizing

Before you use your pump and bottles for the first time, you'll need to sterilize them, and then continue to sterilize at least once a day for most babies under three months old.[3] Ask your pediatrician what's best for your baby.

You can use a bottle sterilizer if you have one, otherwise you can boil all pump and bottle parts on your stovetop: Separate all parts and boil for 5 minutes in a large pot. Remove with tongs and allow to air dry on a clean towel.

Alternatively, you can use the "sanitize," cycle on your dishwasher. Please be aware that some dishwashers get very hot, which can damage smaller pump parts. Place pump and bottle parts on the top dishwasher shelf so that they are as far away from the heat source as possible, and always check for damage after washing.

Please Note: *This is all just general advice—always follow the manufacturer's directions for sterilizing your pump and bottle parts.*

Washing

Wash your pump parts and bottles after every use in hot soapy water. Take all pieces apart and use a bottle brush reserved for baby feeding equipment. Rinse well and leave to air dry on a clean towel. You can also use a dishwasher, but my warning above about very hot dishwashers also applies here.

What Else Do I Need Besides My Pump?

- You may need larger or smaller flanges, depending on the size of your nipples.
- You'll need to replace pump parts per the manufacturer's recommendation, so make sure you have spares on hand. (Not replacing parts can impact the pump's effectiveness and may drop your milk supply.)
- You'll need milk storage bags if you plan on freezing pumped milk.
- You'll need a pump bag and cooler pack if you'll be moving your pump and milk around.
- Some parents who have trouble getting comfortable put nipple butter or coconut oil on their nipples to help decrease friction.
- While a pumping bra is not technically necessary, it's a wonderful convenience if you are going to be pumping multiple times a day. Ask your friends, family, and social media for recommendations.

Now that you've got your pump, let's learn how to use it.

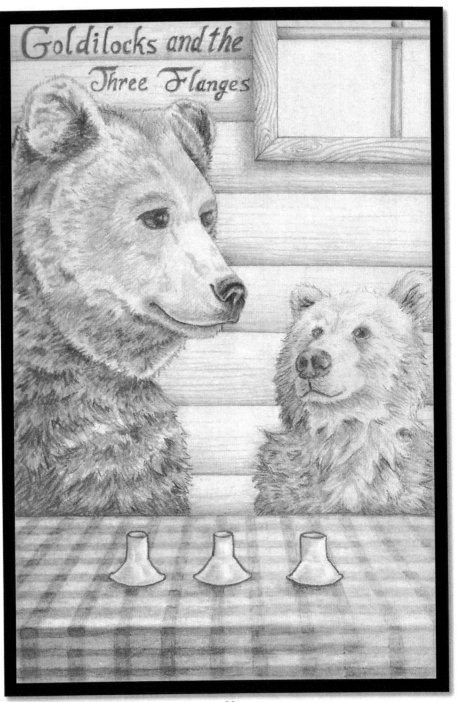

CHAPTER TWO:
HOW DOES MY PUMP WORK...AND WHEN DO I START?

*A*ll pumps work by imitating a baby's sucking pattern. Pumps are really just "robot babies," tagging in for human babies. To make learning more fun, we're going to stop thinking of your pump as a strange and complicated machine and start thinking of it as "Pumpy," your robot baby.

We'll start by reviewing how a baby works to make milk flow, and then learn how you can get Pumpy to do the same.

How the Baby Works

Hungry babies start their feeding at the breast/chest by using a quick suck called a "stimulating suck," to trigger the milk flow. Once the milk is flowing, the baby changes to a slower suck that they use to drink. This slower suck is called a "nutritive suck." When the milk slows down or stops a few minutes into the feeding (this is normal), the hungry baby switches back to that stimulating/quicker suck to make more milk come. This stimulation triggers another letdown of milk at which point they move back to the slower, drinking suck once more. The baby continues feeding like this, switching back and forth between faster and slower sucking, until they are satisfied.

How the Pump Works

All electric pumps have two functions: speed and suction. To make Pumpy imitate an impatient hungry baby, start your pump on a higher speed (your pump may call the higher speed "stimulation" or "massage" mode) and mild suction. When your milk starts to flow, switch modes from fast to slow (your pump may call the slower speed "expression" mode), and increase your suction, to make Pumpy imitate the drinking baby's slower, deeper pull.

On most pumps, there is a button that controls the speed mode. Many pumps automatically switch from fast to slow mode at the two-minute mark, as the pump assumes your milk is flowing by this point. But if your milk starts to flow *before* the two-minute mark, go ahead and press the speed mode button to manually move into slow mode. There's no need to wait.

For the rest of the pumping session, make Pumpy switch back and forth between faster and slower speeds, just like a baby does. As your milk flows, push the button to make Pumpy pull more slowly, and as your milk slows, push the button again to make Pumpy pull more quickly. Some pumps allow you to make adjustments to the rate of speed. You can experiment each time you pump, and fine tune your speed for maximum efficiency.

Now let's talk about suction.

As your milk starts to flow, and you slow down the speed, start increasing the pump's suction. While you may think that cranking the suction all the way up will help you get more milk more quickly, this is not usually the case. Too high a suction may cause pain, and pain can cause *less* milk to flow.[4] You'll need to figure out your own personal suction sweet spot. To do this, turn the suction up gradually. Does it hurt? No? Go up a little more. Does it hurt now? No? Keep going up. At some point, it WILL start to hurt. When it does, turn your suction back down to the last setting where you felt comfortable. This is your highest level of comfort. It's okay to keep your suction at this level for the rest of your session, as long as it remains comfortable.

Now that you understand the mechanics of your pump, we need to make sure it's fitting you well. A good flange fit is critical to effective pumping.

Flanges: Size Matters

Flanges are the part of the pump you hold to your breasts/chest. The flange needs to fit your nipple just right to get the most milk possible.

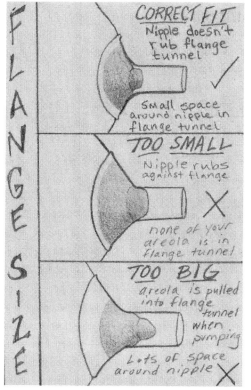

When the flange is just right, your nipple moves freely in and out of the flange, with just a little space around it. You should feel a pull-tug sensation, but no pain. You should see milk flowing within about two minutes and feel pretty empty after about 15.

When the flange is too small, your nipple rubs up against the inside tunnel of the flange in an uncomfortable way.

When the flange is too big, you'll see a large space around your nipple and feel the pump pulling uncomfortably on your areola.

If you're using a flange that is too big or small, you probably won't see much milk, and may still feel somewhat full at the end of a 15-minute pumping session. While you should compare your nipple to the flange opening before you use your pump for the first time, pumping for a few minutes is the best way to know you are using the right size.

If you can tell you're going to have a fit issue just by looking, go ahead and get a different size. Know that it's normal to have nipples that are not the same size and using a different sized flange on each breast is common. Trying a few different sizes to see which ones work best for you is a great strategy.

Ultimately, if pumping is comfortable, and you feel like your pump works well to drain your breasts, you can feel confident you're using the right size.

Please Note: *Your flange size has nothing to do with your breast/chest or areola size. It's all about the nips.*

Now that you understand the basics of your pump, let's move on to when you should start using it, and what a typical pumping session looks like.

I'm often asked,

"Can I Start Pumping Before My Baby Arrives?"

I'm going to answer this question with another question, "What makes you *want* to pump during pregnancy?" The most common answer I hear is rooted in anxiety and sounds something like, "Just in case I don't make enough."

Because I hear it so often, I want to take a moment and explore this belief of "I'm not sure I'll make enough." If you are in good health, having a low-risk pregnancy, and educated about milk making—the odds are fantastic that you'll make plenty of milk. So where is your doubt coming from? I wonder if you're a bit like me and the "I'm not sure I'm enough" feelings aren't just showing up around milk making, but in other areas of your life as well? Anxiety around "not being good/smart/pretty/*whatever* enough" is common, and it makes sense that this anxiety could worsen during pregnancy, when you're getting bombarded with advice for how to be "the best" parent possible. It's stressful!

If you're feeling a little overwhelmed about prepping for parenthood, adding pumping to your pregnancy "to-do" list isn't going to help matters. And as you'll learn in a bit, pumping during pregnancy doesn't typically yield much milk anyway (which makes some anxious parents even *more* anxious when they think there's something wrong with their milk supply).

To lower anxiety levels, instead of trying to express milk, I recommend:

- Talking to supportive loved ones about your worries.
- Making a "gratitude list" of everything that's going well.
- Joining a pregnancy and new parent support group.
- Working with a lactation consultant to create an individualized baby-feeding plan.
- Meeting with a counselor.

General anxiety about not making enough seems to be the most common response to the question, "What makes you want to pump while pregnant?" but let's consider some other reasons.

Many parents start pumping prenatally because social media has led them to believe they're supposed to fill up their freezer with milk, and they're trying to get a head start on this. But the majority of parents don't need to "stock-pile" milk (you'll learn why in Chapter Four), and they wouldn't be able to during pregnancy even if they tried, as pregnancy hormones prevent your milk supply from increasing until the baby is born. This is because your body is super smart and knows when to grow your baby (when the baby is inside) and when to feed your baby (when the baby is outside).

While you are pregnant, your pregnancy hormones (estrogen and progesterone) are switched "on" and running the show, and they force your lactation hormones (prolactin and oxytocin) into the "off" position. If you try to express milk, you'll probably get a few drops of colostrum, but never much more than that. Most parents who are expressing prenatally are doing a lot of work for what usually results in a very small amount of milk.

The only way to throw your lactation hormonal switch "on" is to deliver your baby. When the placenta leaves your body, it takes with it your pregnancy hormones, and only then will your lactation hormones be able to "come online" and increase your supply in response to breast/chest stimulation.

Medical Conditions

Because we don't live in the Fairy Tale World, there are of course situations where babies need extra milk after birth. Babies who are born prematurely, have low blood sugar, or who are small or large for their gestational age are more likely to need a supplement.[5,6] (But many do just fine without one!)

If you or your baby have been diagnosed with a medical condition and you are thinking about prenatal pumping, ask your healthcare provider if this is a safe option for you. When you stimulate your nipples, you release the hormone oxytocin, which contracts both milk-making cells *and* uterine cells. This doesn't seem problematic for low-risk pregnancies,[7] but depending on your circumstances, your doctor may advise against it.

If you decide to try and express colostrum, know that because it is thick and sticky, you might get more out with your hands than with the pump. The pregnant parents I've worked with who collect colostrum typically hand express twice a day, for about 10 minutes per session. They collect the drops of colostrum with a small syringe (1–3 ml) and store them in the freezer.

If you or your baby are facing a medical condition—but you feel uncertain about prenatal expression, have been advised not to do so, or you are struggling to express, know that it's completely okay if you don't bring frozen colostrum with you to the hospital. Once your baby is born and your lactation hormones are switched "on," your body will move into milk-making mode. Keep your baby skin-to-skin as much as you can and nurse them whenever they are hungry. If they end up needing a supplement, hand express and/or pump for about ten minutes after most feedings and feed the baby any colostrum you collect. If you come up short, the hospital will give you donor milk or formula to fill in the gaps until your supply increases.

And if you are separated from your baby, start pumping as soon as you can to get your supply off to a strong start (pg. 73).

The Takeaway on Pumping While Pregnant?

My general recommendation is that there is no need to express milk when you're pregnant. Even if you or your baby are facing a medical concern, it's rarely something you *have* to do. Keep life as simple as possible: Learn about lactation, develop a feeding plan, and cultivate confidence in your body. Then sit back, relax, and enjoy your baby-free time as much as possible. And if expressing milk prenatally is something you decide you would like to do— work with a lactation consultant to achieve the best results.

Another question I hear often is,

"Should I Start Pumping Right After the Baby is Born?"

If you are planning on exclusively pumping and bottle feeding, the answer is "yes," and you can turn to Chapter Seven, "How Do I Exclusively Pump" to learn more (pg. 73).

If you are planning on exclusively breastfeeding/chestfeeding, and everything is going well, then the answer is "no"—there's no need to pump for the first few weeks.

"Everything going well" means:

- Your baby is latching eight to twelve times every 24 hours.
- The latch doesn't hurt.
- Your baby is getting enough to eat (pg. 127).

When these things are happening, your baby is telling your body exactly how much milk to make through that supply-and-demand system we talked about in the introduction. Pumping is just another form of demand in which Pumpy is asking your body for milk instead of your baby. And when you place more of a demand on your body, whether it's through nursing your baby OR pumping, more supply results.

If you were to start pumping on top of breastfeeding/chestfeeding that's going well, your body would make plenty of milk for your baby and then start making *extra milk* for Pumpy. As we mentioned in the last chapter, having more milk than your baby needs tends to cause problems.

Oversupply

Oversupply Problems for You:

- Your breasts can become painfully full.
- The extra milk can get backed up, causing plugged milk ducts.
- Plugged ducts can turn into a breast infection ("mastitis") if not handled quickly and effectively.

Oversupply Problems for Your Baby:

- Milk tends to flow forcefully, causing coughing, excessive spitting up, gas, fussing and tummy trouble.
- You might see blood or mucous in the baby's diapers.
- The tummy issues can result in an unhappy baby who is difficult to soothe.

- Because drinking from a "milk firehose" can be unpleasant, some babies start to refuse the breast.

As long as things are looking good with latching, I recommend you start pumping around three or four weeks postpartum, when it's time to introduce a bottle.

Around this time most babies have gotten pretty good at breastfeeding/chestfeeding, and they're also open to taking a bottle. Some babies refuse the bottle if it is offered after five weeks of age, and there's no way to tell ahead of time if this might happen to you.

Your First Pumping Session

Prepare Before You Begin:

- Sterilize your pump parts.
- Pick a time once a day to pump that you can be fairly consistent with. Many mothers pump in the morning (when milk making hormones are highest) as they tend to see more volume.
- Try to pump within 15 minutes of the end of your nursing session. In this way, you will be asking your body to make more milk specifically at that feeding time.
- If you pump between feedings, you'll be cutting into the milk that your body is getting ready for the next feeding. This is not the end of the world, but your baby may become frustrated at the feeding following your pumping session, as there will be less milk readily available.

Start Pumping:

Step One: Turn on the pump and set it to a quick speed and lower suction.

Center your nipples in the flanges and gently press them against your breasts/chest to create a seal. You will feel a pull-tug sensation and see your nipples moving. This might feel a little unusual but should not hurt.

Within several seconds to several minutes, your milk should start to flow, or "let down."

Step Two: When you notice your milk flowing, turn the pump's speed down, and the suction up, to create that longer slower pull which imitates a drinking baby. Remember to only turn the suction up to your highest level of comfort.

Step Three: After a few minutes, you'll notice the milk slows down or even stops. This is normal, and happens when a baby is nursing, too. A baby who is still hungry will switch back to that quick suck to send the signal, "I'm still hungry, make more milk!" To imitate the hungry baby, switch your pump back to the faster speed, and leave it there until you see milk flowing again or until the session is over.

Step Four: Continue pumping in this way for about 15 minutes (moms of twins can aim for 25), moving back and forth between faster and slower speeds. When milk is flowing, turn your speed to slow. When little to no milk is flowing, turn your speed to fast. You'll only need to adjust your suction if you're feeling uncomfortable; otherwise, it's okay to leave it alone while you switch back and forth between speeds.

Please Note: *Switching back and forth between speeds is useful when establishing a milk supply or when you're trying to boost it. If you're happy with your supply, it's not necessary to switch back and forth between speeds while you pump.*

When 15 minutes is up, you're done! If milk happens to be flowing quickly at the 15-minute mark, allow it to stop, or at least slow down, before ending your session. 20 minutes should be the maximum time spent pumping for most moms with one baby, and 30 minutes maximum for moms of twins.

There should be some milk in your bottles now. Don't panic if you see less than an ounce. Remember that your body has gotten used to making the perfect amount for your baby alone, and Pumpy is new on the scene. As you repeat your pumping session every day, the pump's increased demand will gradually increase your supply. Within a week of starting a daily pumping routine, you should be collecting about 3–4 ounces total after breastfeeding, which makes a complete bottle feeding for most babies. Moms of twins should aim for 6–8 ounces total, if they would like two full bottles.

If Things Are Not Going Well with Breastfeeding/Chestfeeding

If your plan was to breastfeed/chestfeed, but it's not going well, Pumpy needs to tag in for your baby ASAP.

Things are *not* going well if your baby:

- Is latching less than eight times every 24 hours, latching poorly, or not latching at all.
- Is causing pain when they latch.
- Doesn't produce the expected number of diapers (pg. 127).

If any of the above are true, you'll want to start pumping right away to protect your milk supply, and then reach out for help with latching.

Please Note: *A latch that hurts is: 1.) Causing nipple damage that may become infected. 2.) Not allowing your baby to get their fill of milk. When your nipple is getting compressed (this is where the pain is coming from) the flow of milk is restricted. Think about this like your baby "biting on their straw." 3.) Dropping your supply due to the lowered milk flow. Stop latching if it hurts and start pumping and bottle feeding. This is the best way to protect your milk supply and get your baby fed while you get help.*

A baby is supposed to go to the breast at least eight times every 24 hours. If that's not happening, Pumpy needs to start going to the breast at least eight times every 24 hours. Each pumping session should be 15 minutes of double pumping (25 minutes for twins). Many mothers find that pumping every two to three hours during the day, and every three to four hours at night, with one longer stretch of five to six hours of sleep, works well to get to the total of eight. During the first few weeks while you are building a supply, try not to go longer than six hours between pumping sessions.

Please Note: *Reading Chapter Seven, "How Do I Exclusively Pump?" (pg. 73) will be helpful if you end up temporarily exclusively pumping because latching is not going well.*

If your baby does just an *okay* job of breastfeeding/chestfeeding (which would look like five minutes or less of active sucking), you'll want to tag Pumpy in afterwards to fully drain your breasts and stimulate your supply. Double pumping for 10 minutes after a not-so-great feeding is a good plan.

When You *Choose* to Do Some Pumping

Some parents choose to latch for some feedings and bottle feed pumped milk or formula for others. To maintain a full milk supply you'll need at least eight good breast/chest stimulations every 24 hours between the baby and the pump. Moms of twins also need to hit that total of eight, they'll just be pumping for more minutes each session.

Mixed feeding plans that get in eight breast/chest stimulations:

- Latch your baby six times and pump twice during the day, and then have your partner give two bottles overnight (while you sleep!).
- Pump four times during the day while baby gets bottles at daycare and breastfeed/chestfeed four times in the evening and overnight.
- Latch once in the morning and once at night, and pump and bottle feed for the other six feedings.
- Check out page 98 to read more about ways to incorporate pumping and bottle feeding into your routine.

As you can see, there are many options. And as long as you're hitting that magic number of eight every 24 hours, you can switch back and forth between pumping and nursing whenever you'd like. This prompts the question, "Do I need to pump at the same time the baby is getting the bottle? And the answer is no—as long as you are hitting eight breast/chest stimulations every 24 hours, it doesn't matter *when* they happen. You can stack pumping sessions during the day and get more sleep at night.

And if you can't or don't want to get to eight breast stimulations every day? That's okay! You'll still make milk, but should plan on using formula, too. As a general rule, the less often you pump/breastfeed/chestfeed, the less milk you will get, and the more formula you will need to use.

Please Note: *Many parents who plan to combination feed focus on just nursing their babies for the first two or three weeks. This allows them to become pros at latching. However, you can begin combining feeding methods whenever you'd like, just be sure to check out Chapter Seven, "Exclusive Pumping," (pg. 73) to read up on tips and tricks for expressing milk the first week post-partum, when it can be a little tricky.*

The Super Boob

Almost every client I've ever worked with has asked, "One of my breasts produces way more than the other …is this normal? Yes, it's very normal! In fact, it's extremely rare when both breasts are even-steven. Most pumping parents have one overachieving "super boob," and one lagging "dud boob." The good news is, super boob and dud boob usually make a great team. As long as *together* they're eventually able to produce 3–4 ounces total per pumping session in place of a breastfeed (6–8 ounces total for moms with twins), there's nothing to worry about, and no need to try and pump the dud boob more often to encourage it to "catch up."

Okay, so now you know how to pump. How are you storing your milk? And how much *should* you be storing? Read on, my friend!

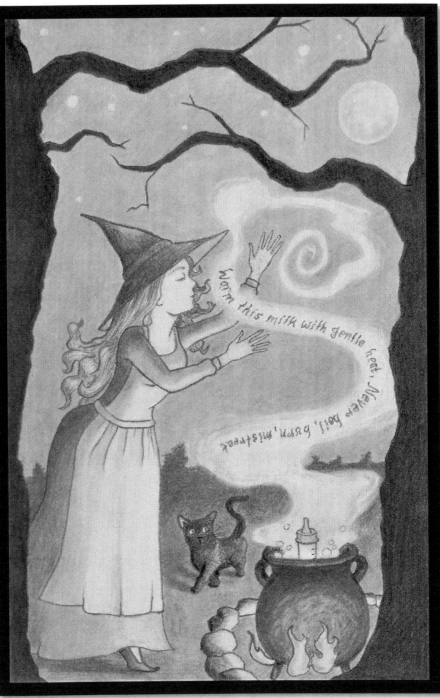

Warm this milk with gentle heat. Never boil, burn, mistreat

CHAPTER THREE:
HOW DO I STORE PUMPED MILK?

The storage, prep and feeding guidelines in this chapter are from the Centers for Disease Control and Prevention (CDC). Visit the CDC's milk storage page[8] for up-to-date information and talk to your pediatrician if you have questions or concerns.

Pumped Milk Storage	
Room temperature	4 hours
Refrigerator	4 days
Freezer	6–12 months
Cooler bag with ice packs	24 hours

Even though pumped milk is technically good for 12 months in the freezer, it's best to use within six. Think about ice cream that's been in your freezer for a year. It's still safe to eat, sure, and retains its *ahem* nutritional value…but it's not very tasty. If you plan on storing pumped milk for longer than six months, consider using a deep freezer, or at the least, put it in the back of your regular freezer, where its temperature will stay more constant.

If you're pumping less milk than you need for a bottle, know that it's okay to combine smaller amounts of milk before freezing. While you'll see varying guidance on this point, my advice is to chill the small amounts of milk separately before combining them and freezing.

Thawing and Reheating Pumped Milk

Defrosting Frozen Milk

- Put frozen milk into the fridge the night before you need to use it.
- Use within 24 hours. (The 24-hour time frame starts when the milk has thawed, and not when you pull it out of the freezer.)
- Never refreeze milk.

Warming Frozen/Cold Milk

- Place the milk in a bowl of warm water or run under warm tap water.
- A bottle warmer is fine, but not necessary.
- Never microwave your milk. Microwaves create hot spots that damage milk and might burn the baby.
- Milk only needs to be lukewarm—think body temperature!
- If your baby will take it, cold milk is totally okay. Just shake it to help mix the fat back in.

Once you start giving a bottle of pumped milk to your baby, the baby needs to finish it within two hours. And if you're using formula, or mixing formula and pumped milk, know that you need to use this milk within one hour after you've started the feed.

Frozen Milk and High Lipase

You may have heard stories of babies who reject freezer milk due to its taking on a strange taste and smell. And while this is not very common, it happens often enough— and creates a big enough problem when it *does* happen—that I want you to be aware. Rejected frozen milk has been described as smelling and tasting "soapy," "metallic," and even "vomit-like" (yuck!).

What's going on here? One theory is that fat molecules in some parent's milk break down more quickly than others due to higher amounts of an enzyme in the milk called *lipase*. Researchers' best guess is that the broken-down fats are responsible for the odd taste and smell.[9] There are alternate theories, but for the purposes of this book, we won't be debating the "why." My goal is to help you create a freezer stash that you know your baby will drink.

The Freezer Test

Freeze a small amount of milk for at least a week, and then offer it to your baby. Even if it smells or tastes different than your fresh milk, "high lipase" milk is safe, and most babies will drink it with no problem. [9] Keep occasionally offering your baby small amounts of more dated frozen milk, to make sure it continues to be palatable over time (as the smell and taste can worsen the longer the milk is frozen).

And what if your baby does refuse the milk? You'll be glad you found out about this sooner rather than later! But whenever you discover the problem, the next section will give you some options for dealing with it.

What if My Baby Refuses My Frozen Milk?

Option One: Opt out of a freezer stash. If you are able to pump for every missed feeding when you work, and are getting 3-4 ounces each time, you should be in pretty good shape to keep up with the milk your baby needs for daycare without storing any (more on this in the next chapter). You'd need to be okay supplementing with formula in the event of a supply dip.

Option Two: Add a drop of *non-alcoholic* vanilla extract to the high lipase milk. There is no evidence on this practice, and you'll see differing opinions. Mine is that there is no known risk in a drop of non-alcoholic vanilla, and if it gets your baby drinking your frozen milk, there is a huge overall benefit. Please check with your baby's pediatrician to see if this option might work for you.

Option Three: Mix some of the frozen milk together with freshly pumped milk. Start with a higher ratio of fresh milk. For example, try a small volume made up of 90% fresh milk and 10% frozen. If baby is willing to take this, you can gradually increase the ratio of frozen milk over time.

Option Four: If all else fails? Human milk banks will usually take high lipase milk. If donating your milk is more appealing than throwing it away, type "human milk banking near me" into your search engine, and you'll find resources to help guide you through the donation process.

Note on Scalding Your Milk: *You might have heard that scalding milk (heating to 170°F) before freezing it eliminates the lipase problem. This seems to work. However, the Academy of Breastfeeding Medicine advises against this practice because we don't have good information on how the nutritional value of the milk changes after it's been heated to 170°F or above.[9] At the very least, we know heat damages beneficial cells, and it stands to reason that the higher the heat, the greater the damage to the milk. If you're pumping to give your baby those beneficial cells but then destroy them by cooking them…I wonder how much it defeats the purpose of pumping? For these reasons, I don't generally recommend scalding your pumped milk.*

Do I Need to Label the Time on My Milk?

You may have heard that you shouldn't use milk you pumped during the day in nighttime bottles, as it might mess with your baby's sleep. While it's true that researchers have found higher levels of "awake and active" hormones in a.m. milk and higher levels of "relaxed and sleepy" hormones in p.m. milk,[10] there is no good evidence about how this might impact babies' sleep, *if at all.*

Many moms pump in the morning and have their partners bottle feed that milk overnight. This has been going on for *decades*, and if it posed a significant sleep issue for the millions of babies involved, I believe we would know about it by now. We only started to worry about the timing of the pumped milk when we were told to, by the media who sensationalized the research.

I have some questions for those stirring up anxiety around "daytime milk" and "nighttime milk" and telling us, "you're doing it wrong!"—Are they worried about what time the cow breast milk they're putting in their coffee was pumped? What about the cow breast milk they give their toddler at bedtime? Shouldn't they be writing a story about how we should be demanding daytime and nighttime infant formula if the time the milk was pumped is so important?

Despite the fact that cows' milk contains a.m. and p.m. hormones much like ours,[11] I've never seen anyone stressing over the cows' pumping times. This leads me to believe that making rules around what *human* milk should be given at what time is just another way to make life more difficult for pumping parents. Therefore, in my opinion, no—you don't need to label the time on your milk, just the date. Make your pumping life as simple and stress-free as possible: Pump whenever it works for you and feed your baby that milk whenever they need it.

Now that you know how to store your milk, let's work out how much you need in your freezer.

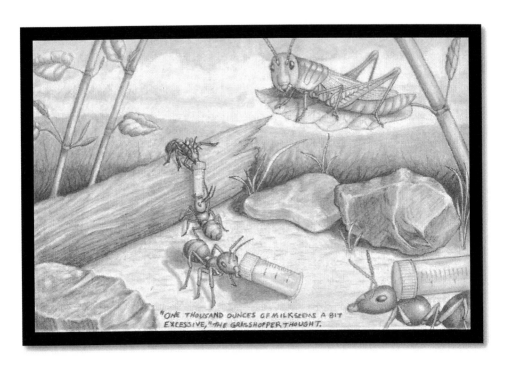

"ONE THOUSAND OUNCES OF MILK SEEMS A BIT EXCESSIVE," THE GRASSHOPPER THOUGHT.

CHAPTER FOUR:

HOW MUCH MILK DO I NEED IN MY FREEZER?

You've seen the pics on social media: freezers bursting with milk, chest freezers in the garage filled to the brim, and videos exclaiming, "How I pump 100 ounces a day!"

Images like these probably make you feel anxious because you don't even have one freezer full of milk let alone *two*, and you wonder how on earth you'll ever be able to pump 100 ounces a day (this is enough milk for triplets, FYI). The good news is, you probably don't need to fill up freezers, nor do you need a triple milk supply (unless you happen to have triplets!).

The amount of milk *you* need to pump every day, and the amount you need in *your* freezer are very specific to you, your baby, and your unique work situation.

Calculate How Much "Daycare Milk" Your Baby Needs

Let's start by figuring out how much milk your baby will need while you're at work. For ease of understanding, let's call this pumped milk, "daycare milk."

Babies between one and six months old eat about 24–32 ounces of milk every 24 hours.[12,13] (After they start solids, their intake may slightly decrease.) This works out to a baby needing roughly 1–1.3 ounces of milk for every hour of the day, and makes it easy to say your baby will need at least as many ounces as hours you are separated. As some babies will need a little more, we'll do some math to get a ballpark range.

To calculate how much "daycare milk" your baby needs:

Hours away from your baby _____

Take the above number and multiply it by 1.3 = _____

- *Example:* *You're going to be away from your baby for 8 hours.*

   Hours away from your baby = __8__. This means you need at least 8 ounces of daycare milk.

   8 ounces × 1.3 = ___10.5___ ounces.

   In this example, you would need to send somewhere between 8–10.5 ounces of milk to daycare every day.

You'll be practicing bottle feeding before you return to work, and so will have a better idea of exactly how much your baby needs by the time you go back.

To get the amount of daycare milk their babies need, most mothers have to pump at work for every missed feeding. For instance, the mother in the example above who is away from her baby for eight hours is probably missing three feeds while she's at work. This means she would likely need to pump three times to get to her goal of 8–10.5 ounces. This is because an average pumping session (in place of a breastfeed/chestfeed) yields about 3–4 ounces total. And 3–4 ounces is (not coincidentally) about how much a baby drinks during an average meal.

Now you know how much milk you need to send to daycare, but how much do you need in your freezer?

Calculate Your Freezer Stash

If you are able to pump at work for each missed feeding like in the previous example, and your output is meeting your baby needs, I've got some great news for you: you don't need much milk in your freezer! When you pump on Monday, that milk goes to daycare on Tuesday. Tuesday's pumped milk goes in for Wednesday, Wednesday's milk goes in for Thursday, Thursday's milk goes in for Friday, and Friday's pumped milk goes into the fridge, to be pulled out on Monday.

In the perfect world of Fairy Tales—this system works flawlessly, and parents don't need any milk in their freezers *at all.*

But of course, we live in the real-life world of *Dairy* Tales, where unfortunately, things are always less-than-perfect. In this reality, babies have growth spurts and occasionally need more than what you were able to pump. Or maybe you leave the pumped milk on the bedstand overnight instead of putting it in the fridge. Or perhaps your partner accidentally knocks over a bottle of milk.

(Whoever said "no crying over spilled milk" obviously didn't pump it themselves.)

Another reason I know we aren't living in a perfect world (but wait, there's more!) is that many mothers see a dip in their supply when they go back to work. This makes sense, as going back to work is a major life transition and therefore pretty darn stressful.

Our imperfect reality means it's a good idea to have a freezer stash, but you don't just want to be squirreling away milk without any rhyme or reason. When you fill up your freezer without a plan, there's a chance that some milk will expire before you can use it, or even worse—you'll run out of room for ice cream.

My general advice for those who can pump at work for every missed feeding is to keep five extra days of daycare milk in the freezer. This is a nice cushion for those times when life doesn't go as planned.

Calculate Your Freezer Stash:

Your baby needs _____ ounces of daycare milk daily.

Take the above number ____ and multiply 5 days,

= _____ ounces (your freezer stash).

- *Example (pulling from the earlier scenario):*

  Your baby needs __8__ ounces of daycare milk daily

  __8__ ounces × 5 days

  = __40__ ounces (your freezer stash).

  In this example, you'll want around 40 ounces of milk in your freezer when you return to work.

If you'll be pumping for every missed feeding like in these examples, you can jump ahead to Chapter Five, "How Do I Build a Freezer Stash," and create your plan.

If you can't (or don't want to) pump for every missed feeding, the next section is for you.

Calculate Your Freezer Stash If You *Don't* Pump at Work

If you aren't pumping at work for every missed feeding, or if you aren't pumping at all, your freezer stash will look different than in the previous example, depending on your situation and goals.

Please Note: *If you want to cut back on your time spent breastfeeding/chestfeeding/pumping when you return to work, be sure and plan ahead to give your body time to adjust (read Appendix A, "Weaning" on page 125).*

Things to consider when planning your freezer stash:

- How many times will you pump at work?
- For how long do you want your baby to get your milk?
- When are you okay with introducing formula, and how much do you want to use?
- Do you want to keep breastfeeding/chestfeeding/pumping at home and wean during your workday? (Yes, this is a thing!)
- How much time are you willing to spend pumping during your maternity leave?

While it's impossible to review every possible option, below are a few common scenarios for parents who don't pump at work for every missed feeding.

Scenario One: No Pumping at Work

If you'd like to breastfeed/chestfeed/pump at home but not pump at work, you can create a freezer stash of pumped milk that's just for daycare. To figure out a freezer stash in this scenario, multiply the daily daycare ounces your baby needs by the number of days you want them fed with just your milk at daycare.

For example, let's say you want your baby to get your milk for three months at daycare after you go back to work. Take those 90 days and multiply them by the 8 ounces of daily daycare milk needed, to get a freezer stash of 720 ounces.

Please Note: *Your baby will need that daycare milk on the weekends, too, as your supply will always be low during the day after you wean back on breastfeeding/chestfeeding/pumping at that time.*

Scenario Two: Some Pumping at Work

In this situation, you are planning to do *some* pumping at work, but not enough to cover every missed feeding. For example, your baby will need to eat three times while you are at work, but you will only be pumping once.

To get your freezer stash— start by multiplying your daily daycare milk number by the number of days you want your baby to get your milk.

Following the previous example, imagine you want your baby to have pumped milk for 90 days after you go back to work. Multiply the 90 days by the 8 ounces of daily daycare milk to get a total of 720 ounces. But 720 isn't your freezer number this time, because you're going to do *some* pumping at work which will reduce the total amount you need in the freezer. Let's pretend you can pump at work once a day, and let's say you pump about 4 ounces during that one pumping session.

The next step is to take that 4 ounces you'll be pumping every day and multiply it by the number of days you want baby getting your milk (in this example 90 days). $4 \times 90 = 360$ ounces you'll be pumping over those three months.

Finally, to determine your freezer stash, subtract the amount of milk you're able to pump, (360 ounces) from the amount of daycare milk you determined your baby needs. In other words, take the 720 ounces your baby needs and subtract the 360 ounces you will be pumping at work, and you'll arrive at needing 360 ounces in your freezer.

Scenario Three: Weaning Before You Return to Work

This option is for parents for who want to be completely dried up when they go back to work but want their baby to continue drinking their milk (both at home and at work).

To get your freezer stash, multiply the number of days you want your baby to get your milk after you return to work by 25 ounces a day (25 ounces is just an average daily intake for exclusively breastfed/chestfed babies; your baby's intake may be higher or lower).

For example, let's imagine you want your baby to get pumped milk for three months after you wean. Take the 90 days you want your baby to get your milk and multiply that by the 25 ounces of pumped milk they need every day, to get a freezer stash of 2,250 ounces. (Now you can see why filling up freezers might make sense for certain parents!)

Who knew you'd need algebra to feed a baby?

Hopefully you found an example similar to your situation, and you can plug your own numbers in to figure out your specific freezer stash.

And hopefully you've come to understand just how specific this number is to you. You absolutely cannot compare yourself to what another parent is doing when talking about a freezer stash.

What if I Don't Want to Pump During my Maternity Leave?

Like we discussed earlier in this chapter, if you're planning to pump at work for every missed feeding, you don't really need much of a freezer stash. Therefore, if you don't feel driven to spend your maternity leave pumping and feeding your freezer, that's okay! If your supply dips when you return to work, you can use some formula to fill in the gaps while your body gets used to the new routine. In these cases, I recommend talking to your pediatrician and introducing some formula a week or two before you go back, to make sure your baby is okay with it.

For those of you facing a large freezer stash number because you *won't* be doing much pumping at work, but you also don't want to spend your entire maternity leave pumping—think about how formula can be incorporated into your plan. Consider how much formula you want to send to daycare every day, and then subtract that amount from the total amount of daycare milk you figured you needed. This should get you a freezer stash number that seems more manageable.

And know that some parents throw the freezer number out the window altogether. I've met many parents who don't pump during their maternity leave, don't pump at work, send formula to daycare, and then continue breastfeeding/chestfeeding/pumping when they're at home. There's no one right way to do this. You get to decide what's best for you.

However much milk you've decided you want in your freezer, you're probably wondering how to get it in there. Keep reading.

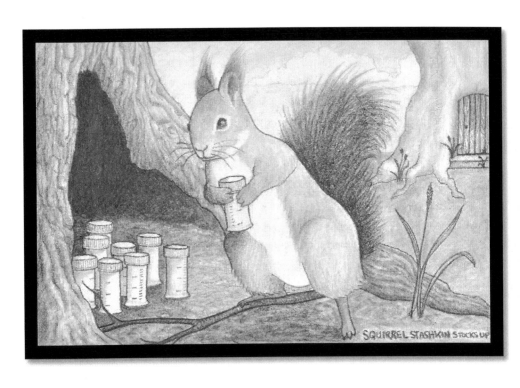

CHAPTER FIVE:
HOW DO I
BUILD A FREEZER STASH?

As we talked about in Chapter Two, as long as breastfeeding/chest-feeding is going well, I recommend you start pumping around three or four weeks postpartum so that you can introduce the bottle. Around the same time, you may want to start creating your freezer stash. In this chapter I'll help you think through how long it's going to take, and what it will entail.

Pumping Once a Day

Pumping once a day *might* work to build your freezer stash. This depends upon how much milk you are able to pump, how often you bottle feed, and how much time you have before returning to work. After a week of pumping once a day after breastfeeding/chestfeeding, you should be getting enough for a full bottle feed (around 3–4 ounces). If you're lucky enough to be pumping more than what your baby is taking, you can freeze any extra. You could also choose to only give an ounce or so in the bottle for practice once a day and stash the rest. Another option would be to keep pumping every day, but only practice bottle feeding every *other* day (which seems to be enough to keep babies happily switching back and forth). This would allow you to build your freezer stash more quickly and without adding extra pumping to your day.

However, many parents use all of the milk from their once-a-day pumping session during their once-a-day bottle feed. These parents will need to add a second pumping session to their day in order to create a freezer stash and/or try "working smarter" to maximize their current pumping efforts (pg. 64).

Pumping Twice a Day (Or More)

If once a day isn't cutting it to feed your freezer, pick a second time of the day where you can pump after breastfeeding. It will take about a week for your supply to increase during this pumping session, and for you to start seeing a consistent amount of milk.

If your freezer stash number is quite large and you are short on time, you might be adding even more pumping sessions to your day. Do this by picking another time you can be consistent with, or alternately you can go rogue with your pumping (next section). Remember that all of this increased pumping will be boosting your overall supply. To avoid engorgement at work, you'll need to gradually wean back down to your desired level before going back.

Please Note: *Your freezer stash isn't more important than your physical, mental and emotional health. If you are pumping more than twice a day in addition to exclusively breastfeeding/chestfeeding, I want you to check in with yourself and your family, to make sure you're feeling calm, balanced, and enjoying parenthood. If you're feeling pressured, stressed, and like you're spending more time with your pump than with your family, consider pulling back on the pumping and planning to use some formula.*

Rogue Pumping

Rogue pumpers find it tricky to follow a consistent schedule, and so pump whenever they can. Sometimes they pump for the full fifteen minutes, sometimes they pump for only five, and sometimes they power pump for an hour. Because it's not a set schedule, the amount of milk pumped per session is unpredictable. But that's okay! Remember that you only need a few ounces for bottle feeding practice a few days a week, and any excess you pump can go in the freezer.

How Long Will It Take to Build my Freezer Stash?

If you're able to pump on a consistent schedule, you can figure out how long it's going to take to build your freezer stash by using the equation below. Give your body a week to adjust to your new pumping routine before doing this math, as it can take that long to see consistent amounts.

Ready for a math quiz?

> *If a mother has been pumping an average of 3 extra ounces a day, and is trying to store 60 ounces total in her freezer, how many days will it take her to complete her freezer stash?*

If you answered, "20 days," you get a gold star!

And if pop quizzes aren't your thing, here's the cheat sheet:

_____ ounces = Your freezer stash goal.

Take the number above and divide it by the _____ ounces you put in your freezer every day.

=_____ days to reach your goal.

- ***Example:*** *The mother in the quiz needed*

   ___60___ ounces for her freezer stash

   (÷) ___3___ ounces she puts in her freezer every day

   = ___20___ days to reach her goal.

53

A Note for Rogue Pumpers: *Because you are pumping different amounts of milk every day, it's pretty difficult to determine how long it's going to take you to build your freezer stash. My advice is to check in on your freezer every week. Depending on how it's looking as your return-to-work date approaches, you may need to consider how formula can fit into your plans.*

If you are feeling pretty good about a plan to pump and build your freezer stash, you can skip over to Chapter Seven and start learning about bottle feeding.

If you feel like your supply is falling short, the next chapter offers some tips on how to make more milk.

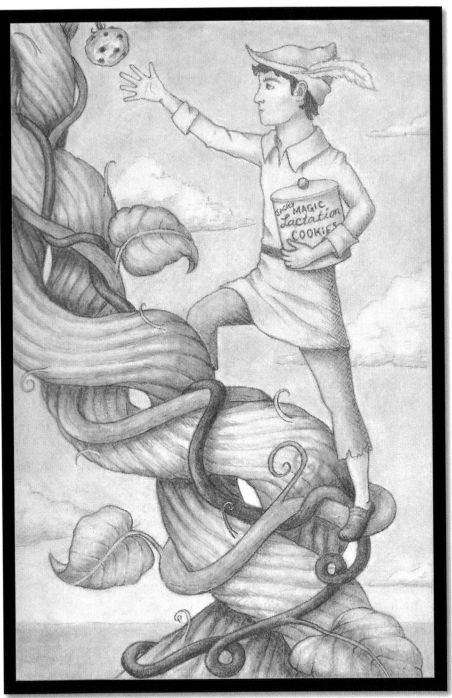

CHAPTER SIX:
HOW CAN I BOOST MY SUPPLY?

In the Fairy Tale World, cookies solve problems: Fighting with your spouse? Eat one chocolate chip cookie apiece, and your love will be restored. Boss demanding too much of your time? Eat three small macadamia nut cookies, and prepare to enjoy some free time. Not pumping enough milk? No worries, just eat one lactation cookie per day, and the rivers of milk will flow.

Sound too good to be true? Sadly, it is. In our real-life Dairy Tale World, cookies are a fun treat, and nothing more.

Well, *almost* nothing more....

Lactation Cookies and Other "Milk-Boosting" Foods

Lactation cookies (and shakes, bars, brownies, etc.) DO contain a few ingredients known as "galactagogues." Galactagogues are foods that may boost supply a tiny bit,[14] as long as the mother is also regularly breastfeeding/chestfeeding or pumping. Because every culture in the world has a different list of foods they believe help make milk, the list of alleged galactagogues is quite lengthy. Some common foods you'll see linked to lactation across cultures include oats, brewer's yeast, dark leafy greens, sweet potatoes, fennel, garlic, and flax seeds.

Lactation cookies and other commercially prepared foods marketed as a "milk boosters" generally contain the galactagogues of oatmeal, brewer's yeast, and flax seeds. Even if these ingredients *might* work to increase a milk supply, I wonder if they have any impact at all when present in the small amounts found in a packaged snack? All signs point to "no," although you will hear people swearing up and down that these lactation cookies are helping. So what's really going on? Why is everyone cookie-crazy? Is there any truth to all the hype?

Here are four possible causes for any positive reviews you come across:

1. Some mothers are eating lactation cookies from day one because they think they *have to* in order to make milk. As they watch their supply increase over the first week, they post on social media, "wow, these cookies really work!!!" But as long as a mother is regularly breastfeeding/chestfeeding or pumping, her supply quickly increases during the first few days, as that's just how milk-making works. The cookie had nothing to do with this natural supply-and-demand system.

2. Parents with a low supply learn that they need to pump more to see an increase. After a day or two of pumping and not seeing any results, they get desperate and buy lactation cookies. On day three, they continue to pump, and eat tons of cookies. On day four, they see an increase in their milk supply and swear it was the cookies that made the difference. What they didn't know was that it normally takes about three to five days of consistent pumping to see an increase in supply, and so once again, the cookie connection was just a coincidence.

3. I don't know about you, but when I eat cookies, my body relaxes into a state of bliss. And while being in a relaxed state doesn't produce more milk directly, it might help milk that's already there flow a little easier. And if a little more milk flows, then a little more milk will be made to replace it. And so there may be something to the

idea that a cookie that helps a parent relax is *indirectly* boosting their milk supply. But of course, there are other ways to relax that don't involve cookies, that might similarly boost supply.

4. The placebo effect is a force to be reckoned with when considering the cookie question. When a mother deeply *believes* that a lactation cookie (or a cup of tea, or a daily back massage, or wearing her lucky bra) will help her make more milk, she might actually make more milk—just through the belief alone. We don't really understand how the placebo effect works, but the evidence clearly shows that it does.[15] In any event, success in this case is somehow related to the power of positive thinking, and not the cookie itself.

What's the takeaway on cookies and galactagogues?

For parents who are doing everything they can to boost supply (i.e. following the tips found later in this chapter), adding healthy foods categorized as galactagogues to their diet can't hurt and might help. Instead of snacking on cookies though, consider eating a bowl of oatmeal sprinkled with ground flax seeds and brewer's yeast. In this way, you can take in more of the alleged milk-boosting ingredients, without the extra sugar and calories found in the cookies. You'll also be out less money, as those packaged lactation cookies aren't cheap.

All of that being said…if you like the cookies, eat the cookies! While they are probably not doing much for your supply, they're not hurting anything. And if they are making your baby-feeding life more pleasurable, this is a great reason to keep them in the mix.

To conclude this section on foods—despite what you're reading on social media, know that there is nothing you *have* to eat in order to make milk. Do your best to eat a variety of nutritious foods every day, to keep yourself as healthy as possible. When you are in a good state of health (mental, physical and emotional), your milk making efforts will go as smoothly as possible.

Mother's Milk Teas and Herbal Supplements

Teas, drinks, and supplements marketed as "milk-boosters" generally contain herbs regarded as galactagogues, and just like with the milk-boosting foods list, you'll find a long list of herbs linked to lactation as well. Common herbal galactagogues include moringa, fenugreek, alfalfa, goat's rue and blessed thistle. These herbs might increase milk volume by a small amount,[14] as long as the parent is also regularly breastfeeding/chestfeeding or pumping.

As far as any version of a "mother's milk" tea goes, you'd have to drink several cups of tea over the course of the day to notice any benefit. But drinking tea can be relaxing, and so just like with the cookies, the relaxing effects of tea might end up indirectly boosting your supply, regardless of your intake. If you don't like the taste of the tea or want to be more certain about the amount of an herb you are taking in, you can take these same milk-boosting herbs in capsule or tincture form.

Please talk to your health care provider and a lactation consultant before taking any milk-boosting supplement. Some of the herbs that work to give a slight boost to one person's milk supply may cause a decrease in another's, depending on their medical histories. Some herbs interfere with the absorption of medications and may cause allergic reactions. Remember that just because a product is "natural" does not mean it is harmless.

Hydration and Special Drinks

You may have heard that drinking gallons of water or special drinks will help boost your supply. And these liquids DO have the potential to boost your supply...*but only if you were dehydrated to begin with.* A fun fact is that when you're caring for a newborn 24/7, it's not that hard to become dehydrated, and I think this is how some of the "drink THIS to boost supply" messages get started on social media.

For example, imagine I'm not taking great care of myself after my baby arrives (true story), and I become a little dehydrated. My milk supply dips, so I search online and see over and over, "Betty's Blue Drink will boost your supply!" I buy a case of Betty's Blue Drink and start chugging. And lo and behold, my supply comes back up over the next few hours. Could you blame me for thinking, "Wow, that Betty's Blue Drink really DOES increase supply!"? And you wouldn't be surprised if I went online and added my own testimonial about Betty's Blue Drink.

But what if I had just chugged water to rehydrate instead of Betty's Blue Drink? Would my supply still have come back up? The answer is "no," because the blue dye in Betty's Blue Drink has magical properties that miraculously increase milk supply.

Just kidding!

The answer is "yes"— As my body was rehydrated by drinking plain old (free) tap water, my supply would have come back up.

So how much water do you need to drink? Because every lactating parent is different, and making a different amount of milk, there's not a specific amount…but you *will* likely be feeling thirstier than when you were pregnant, and so need to pay attention to your body. My advice is, "drink to thirst," which means that when you feel thirsty, just drink until you're not thirsty anymore. Keep a water bottle next to where you breastfeed/chestfeed/pump and remember to drink from it every time you sit down.

And so sadly, it seems as though the "magic beans" methods of increasing supply (foods, drinks, supplements) are not the easy fix we all wish they were. Which leads you to ask, "so what *really* works, then, to boost milk volume?"

Working Harder

The most effective way to increase your supply is to breastfeed/chestfeed or pump more often. No one likes this answer, as pumping is way less fun than eating cookies, but it is THE answer. The principle of milk making is key here: The more milk your baby or pump takes, the more milk your body makes. Remember that you need to hit that magic number of eight breast stimulations every 24 hours (pg. 9) between the baby and the pump to even be *expecting* a full supply, and that nursing and pumping need to be comfortable and effective for this to work.

If you're falling short of eight, try the "working harder" tips below, and you should notice an increase in your supply within about a week. And if you're already at that magic number of eight and not seeing results? Skip ahead to the "Working Smarter" section in this chapter to troubleshoot and maximize your current efforts.

Please Note: *Eight as the "magic number" is a "One Size Fits Most" situation: eight breast stimulations a day work well to create a full milk supply for MOST mothers…but not ALL. There will be some parents who need a little less stimulation to create a full supply, and some who need a little more. If you are breastfeeding/chestfeeding 5 times a day, pumping twice, and this is working to keep your baby fed, then seven is your magic number. If you find that eight good breast stimulations just aren't cutting it, your magic number might be nine. If you're at a nine and **still** falling short…I'd encourage you to work with a lactation consultant, to explore what else might be hindering your supply.*

Tips for Working Harder:

- **Add an extra pumping session to your day.** The more minutes of pumping you add to your day, the more of an increase in your supply. A full pumping session is ideal, but if you only have five or ten minutes to pump instead of the full 15, go for it! Every minute helps.

  Please Note: *Be as consistent as possible with the timing of this added pumping session, to get a good idea of how much your supply is increasing over time.*

Also Note: *Sometimes the pumping works to boost supply…but then your baby ends up drinking the extra milk! In this case, you might not see an increase in your pumping volume. You'll know you're making more though, as your breasts/chest will feel fuller, and your baby will be more satisfied after nursing.*

- **Nurse your baby more often.** Whenever they seem willing to have a little snack, pop your baby on the boob. Great times to try this are right before they fall asleep and right as they wake up. Dream feeds work great to get in a few extra minutes of nursing, too! (A "dream feed" is when you gently wake your sleeping baby and bring them to the breast/chest for a few minutes of nursing.)

- **Let your baby "use you as a pacifier."** Contrary to this popular saying, your baby is not USING you. Babies aren't capable of this kind of manipulation. (Toddlers are another story!) Offering your baby comfort through your body doesn't constitute a "bad habit" any more than giving a big, long hug to an older child does. If you have a low supply and a baby who likes to hang out on the boob, consider allowing them to do this whenever it works for you, as it's an easy (and snuggly) way to boost supply.

- **Use your soft silicone pump in your downtime.** While not as effective as an electric pump, this pump is great when you have a few spare minutes of lounging time. Consider buying two and wearing them at the same time.

- **Warm up your breasts/chest and your flanges** right before you nurse your baby or pump. Check out the breast warmers on the market, or just use a warm washcloth. To heat your flanges, run them under warm water.

- **Try "power pumping."** The idea here is to have Pumpy act like a human baby who is cluster feeding:
  - Pump for 20 minutes.
  - Rest for 10 minutes.
  - Pump for 10 minutes.
  - Rest for 10 minutes.
  - Pump for 10 minutes to finish out the hour.

Sometimes it's difficult to come up with the extra time needed to "work harder" at boosting supply, which leads us to "working smarter."

Working Smarter

The idea behind "working smarter" is to enhance the time you are already spending nursing/pumping, to make it as effective as possible.

Working Smarter While Breastfeeding/Chestfeeding

- **Breastfeed/chestfeed skin-to-skin and hold your baby skin-to-skin as often as you can.** This boosts oxytocin levels, which helps your milk flow more easily. Skin-to-skin holding also encourages babies to latch more often, which is bonus breast stimulation. A baby carrier or wrap is a great way to easily spend skin-to-skin time with your baby.

- **Make sure your baby has as deep latch.** A baby with a deep latch removes the most milk possible.

- **Use gentle breast/chest compressions.** When your milk slows down a few minutes into the feeding (babies will let you know because they suck less vigorously or start falling asleep), gently compress your breast/chest to keep the milk flowing. As described in my book "Breastfeeding 101: Prepare for the Suck":

When your baby starts to slow down on their sucking, give your breast/chest a gentle squeeze and watch their response. If they start showing wide rhythmic sucking again, hold that squeeze until they've stopped. Then move your hand to a new spot. Wait for your baby to start sucking again, and gently squeeze again. Once they no longer respond to the squeezes, you'll know that side is pretty empty and it's time to switch.

- **Offer both sides.** This may seem obvious, but I have worked with mothers who think that one breast per feeding is enough, and then wonder why their supply is dropping. Some parents with a very strong milk supply can get away with using one breast per feeding, but this is not the norm. Most babies will take one full breast and usually half of the other, but some will need to drain both.

- **Switch sides more than once.** If your baby has emptied both breasts but is still looking hungry, try putting them back on the first side before giving them a bottle. Your body makes milk on the spot during a breastfeeding/chestfeeding session, and so while your baby was nursing on the second breast, the first one was starting to fill up again. Your baby might go back to that first side for only a minute or two, but every minute counts!

- **Use your soft silicone pump while breastfeeding/chestfeeding.** Wear it on your opposite breast while your baby is nursing. Switch sides when baby switches.

Working Smarter While Pumping

- **Use your hands when pumping.** A baby at the breast uses both compression and suction. Adding gentle compressions to the pump's suction better imitates the baby and so tends to yield more milk. There's no right or wrong here, just gently squeeze and press around your breasts in a way that doesn't mess up the pump's attachment. If you see more milk flowing as you compress, hold that gentle squeeze until the flow slows down. Then move your hand to a new spot and repeat. At the time of this writing (2022), Stanford University Medicine's website features a helpful "hands-on" pumping video to help you learn this skill.[16]

- **Be sure your flanges fit.** If your flanges are the wrong size, you will probably not be able to fully drain your breasts.

- **Replace pump parts** as often as recommended by the manufacturer, as not doing so can drop your supply over time.

- **Use your pump most effectively.** Switch back and forth between fast and slow speeds as your milk ebbs and flows.

- **Pump more often in the morning.** Milk-making hormones are highest for most parents in the morning and decline throughout the day. For this reason, you'll probably see more milk when you pump at 7 a.m. than when you pump at 7 p.m.

- **Try lactation massagers.** These small devices warm up and gently vibrate to help milk flow more easily. (Your hands can pretty much do the same thing, but get tired—whereas these gadgets don't!)

- **Look at photos or videos of your baby** and hold their blanket when you pump. These things might help you feel a bit more relaxed and snuggly, which can help your milk flow.

- **Change up the stimulation.** Start your 15-minute pumping session with eight minutes of double-electric pumping. Then move to a single-sided pump for two minutes on each side, using your free hand to gently massage the side being pumped. For the remaining three minutes, hand express on both sides (pg. 74).

- **Pump even when no milk is flowing.** If your milk stops flowing at the 10-minute mark, keep the pump running for another five minutes in "fast" mode. The increased stimulation is boosting your milk-making hormones. These hormones are "calling in an order"

66

for more milk, and after a few days, you should start to see more milk output during this time.

- **Try an essential oil diffuser.** Smelling something pleasant can help you take deeper breaths and relax, which may help milk flow more easily.

What if you're doing all of the above, and your supply hasn't budged within a week (remember it may take this long to see results)? It may be time to stop trying harder and start trying softer.

Trying Softer

Having a new baby is beautiful, magical, wonderful – and also a major life transition. It's normal to feel like you don't have enough hands, you don't have enough time, you don't have enough help. When baby feeding is not going as planned, stress levels can easily start to snowball.

High levels of stress hormones can block oxytocin[17], the hormone that allows milk to flow freely. If less milk flows, the baby will take less, and over time, your supply will likely drop. And then if you add in the stress of working SO HARD to bring it back up... it may drop even further. If this situation sounds familiar, I want you to take a step back, take a deep breath, and consider "trying softer."

Relaxing as much as you can in general as well as relaxing your efforts to make milk can paradoxically work to increase your supply. But as you'll see in the first tip, part of trying softer involves shifting your perspective, and moving away from the idea that, "the more milk I produce, the better I'm doing." I want you to feel good, and happy, and like you're doing a good job, regardless of the amount of milk you make.

Tips for Trying Softer

- **Change your definition of success.** From now on, success has nothing to do with what your baby is eating or how many ounces of milk your body makes:

  If your baby is fed and loved, and you are feeling healthy and balanced (always a work in progress!)—you are rocking it, period.

- **Remind yourself often that your baby loves you.** They think you are the most amazing human on the planet, and nothing compares to you.

- **Ask for help** with your baby, your other children, your pets, your housework, etc. Most people in your life would love to help. If you don't have friends or family nearby, consider hiring someone temporarily.

- **Sleep as often as you can.** Have someone give your baby a bottle so you can sleep for a longer stretch. If the bottle has pumped milk in it, magnificent. If it has formula in it, fantastic. As long as you are getting in about eight breast stimulations every 24 hours, one bottle of formula is not going to ruin your milk supply. And getting more than a two-hour stretch of sleep may very well help it.

- **Eat as balanced a diet as you can manage**, and be sure to include foods that make you smile.

- **Continue taking your prenatal (or multi) vitamin.** This fills in any nutritional gaps.

- **Drink to thirst.** Keep a bottle of water wherever you sit to nurse/pump…and remember to drink it!

- **Relax and treat yourself.** I want you to seriously answer this question: When was the last time you enjoyed yourself? It's time…!

  Treating yourself might include:
    o Listening to your favorite songs
    o Taking a bubble bath
    o Watching funny cat videos
    o Taking a yoga class
    o Dancing in your living room
    o Eating ice cream
    o Having a girls' night out

  Heck, do all of these in one day and kiss your stress goodbye.

  Please Note: *Taking a break from your baby is not "selfish." On the contrary, balancing your physical, emotional, and mental health is a super healthy habit, one that allows you to show up as the best version of yourself. And when you are in balance, your milk supply will be as strong as possible.*

- **Enjoy a glass of wine.** If you pump or nurse before that (5-ounce) glass of wine and wait at least two hours before feeding/pumping, the alcohol will be cleared from your bloodstream and therefore out of your milk. If wine is not your thing, one 12-ounce beer, or one 1-ounce shot is okay, too. (Check out the CDC's page on alcohol and breastfeeding[18] for the details and talk to your health care provider.)

- **Use your imagination.** Visualize your breasts filling, milk leaking, and your baby looking full and relaxed. Imagine this as often as you can, and especially in the moments before you fall asleep. In the stage between awake and asleep, your conscious and subconscious are more connected, and a self-hypnosis of sorts seems possible. While we currently only have limited research on these kinds of techniques,[19] there is plenty of positive anecdotal evidence, it costs nothing, and so definitely can't hurt, and might help.

- **Have a heart-to-heart with your baby.** Tell them how it's going, how you're feeling, and how much you love them. The baby may or may not understand (I think they do!), but in any event, talking to them like this might help you feel more relaxed.

- **Use a sixty-second meditation before pumping:**

  o 20 seconds—Close your eyes, take three deep breaths, and feel the tension leave your body every time you exhale.
  o 20 seconds—Imagine holding your baby. Feel their weight in your arms. Breathe in their scent. Picture your baby smiling up at you, loving you.
  o 20 second affirmation—Saying this out loud is best if you can:

  "I am doing my best to nourish my baby through pumping. I am thankful for this time.
  I honor my body for providing milk and am grateful for every drop that comes...but I also know my worth as a mother is not measured in ounces.
  I am the best mother for my baby just as I am.
  I am enough."

The "trying softer" techniques are great mental health practices in and of themselves. Feeling calmer and more centered, regardless of where your milk supply is at, is reason enough to continue trying softer.

Medications

If you have tried everything in this chapter, and nothing is working to increase your supply, talk to a lactation consultant and your health care provider to explore what else can be done. Bloodwork can help identify if a hormonal imbalance is at play. If your levels of prolactin are low, you may consider trying a prescription medication that has the side-effect of boosting this milk-making hormone. The two most common medications used by parents trying to increase their milk supply are Metoclopramide (Reglan) and Domperidone (Motilium). Your health care provider can discuss the benefits and risks specific to you.

If you are ready to move on to bottle feeding, turn to page 85. If you're looking to learn more about exclusive pumping, keep right on reading.

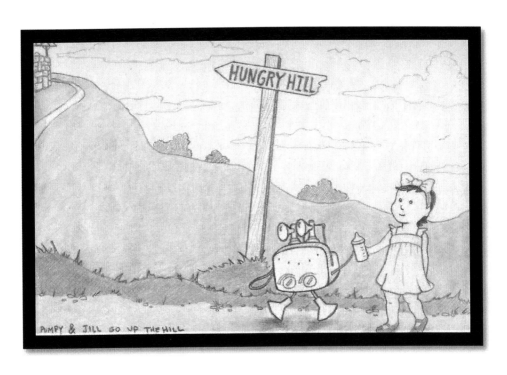

CHAPTER SEVEN:
How Do I Exclusively Pump?

E xclusively pumping parents don't latch their babies to the breast/chest, but rather pump and bottle feed. If you are considering exclusive pumping, this chapter will help you establish and maintain a full supply of milk through pumping alone.

To get your milk supply off to a strong start you'll need Pumpy, the robot baby, to imitate a human baby as closely as possible. A baby goes to the breast within the first hour of life to get those milk-making hormones flowing, and so Pumpy should be going to the breast within the first hour of life, too (or as soon as possible). A baby goes to the breast at least eight times every 24 hours to establish a full milk supply, and so Pumpy should be going to the breast at least eight times every 24 hours, too.

While you are in the hospital, there are some benefits to using their multi-user, "hospital grade" pump which works well to establish a milk supply. As a bonus, when you use their pump, you'll have access to different sized flanges should you need them, colostrum cups that screw on to the pump flanges (more on that below), and maybe even a hand pump. I recommend bringing your single-user, double electric pump to the hospital and comparing it's effectiveness to the multi-user. If you feel like the hospital's pump is doing a noticeably better job of making your colostrum flow, consider renting one, if only for a week or two, to establish your milk supply. Once you feel good about your supply, you can start using your single-user pump to maintain it.

Pumping and Hand Expressing Colostrum

Colostrum is the milk your body makes during pregnancy; it is ready and waiting when your baby is born. It's thick and sticky, and while easily removed by a baby (who uses both compression and suction), colostrum can be more difficult to remove with the pump alone (which uses only suction). Experiment to see how much colostrum you get with your hands versus the pump.

If you're like most mothers, you'll find that your hands work better, but this is literally "manual labor," which is tiring! Luckily, Pumpy never gets tired, and so while your pump is typically not as good at removing colostrum, it is still worth using for the easy breast stimulation. For these reasons, I recommend combining pumping and hand expression for the first few days.

Please Note: *If the pump is working well to express your colostrum, there's no need to hand express.*

As we've already covered how to use a pump (pg. 29), let's learn how to hand express.

How to Hand Express

Seeing hand expression in action tends to be a far better teaching tool than just reading about it. At the time of this writing (2022), Stanford University Medicine's website features a hand expression video that you may find helpful.[20]

1. **Step One:** Wash your hands and have a small container ready (spoon, medicine cup, colostrum cup, or syringe) to catch the drops of milk. Take a few deep breaths and try to relax as much as possible.

2. **Step Two:** Place your pointer finger and thumb about two inches back from your nipple.

3. **Step Three**: Press back into your chest wall, towards your ribcage, and gently roll your fingers together. Then release, keeping your fingers in place.

    Please Note: *You are not dragging your finger and thumb over your skin towards your nipple. Your finger and thumb are staying pretty much in the same place while they press back and then roll towards the nipple.*

4. **Step Four:** Repeat step three, in a rhythmic motion, until you see drops of milk appear on your nipple: Press back into your chest wall, compress by rolling your fingers together, release, and then repeat.

    Please Note: *It can take a few minutes of hand expression to see drops of colostrum. This is normal.*

5. **Step Five:** Once you no longer see milk, move your finger and thumb to a new place on your breast. Press back into your chest wall, compress by rolling your fingers together, release, and then repeat.

The above is just one way to hand express. Experiment to see what works best for you.

Milk Volume on Day One and Two

Whether you are pumping and/or hand expressing, when you express milk on day one and two, it's normal to see only teaspoon-sized amounts (2–10 ml) of colostrum after each session. (For your reference, a baking teaspoon holds 5 ml.) If you were collecting these drops in the 5-ounce bottles (150 ml) that come with your pump, you'd wind up with two tiny puddles at the bottom, which are hard to get out. Ask the hospital for some colostrum cups and small syringes. Colostrum cups are 1-ounce (30 ml) containers that you can attach to your pump and hand express into. Because they're small, it's easy to remove the colostrum at the end of your session. You can use a syringe to pull up the expressed milk, and then finger feed it to your baby.

Finger Feeding

For the small amounts of colostrum you'll express on day one and two, a feeding syringe often works better than a bottle. The hospital staff can help you when the time comes, but here are a few tips to get you familiar with the finger-feeding process. This is ideally a two-person job, one person to hold the baby, and the other to do the feeding:

- Hold your baby in an upright position.

- Tap their lips with a clean finger. When they open, gently and slowly slide your finger, pad side up, into the roof of their mouth. Your finger touching their palate will trigger their suck reflex.

- After they start sucking, tuck the syringe into the corner of their mouth, and give an **extremely gentle** push on the plunger, as the milk often flows more quickly than you expect. The goal is for only a few drops of milk to come out with each push, so the baby doesn't get overwhelmed with too much too fast, or choke.

- As the milk flows, you'll see and feel your baby switch from a shallower suck to a deeper suck that means they're actively drinking.

- Let them drink for about three to five seconds and then give them a break to breathe. They will likely stop sucking for a few seconds.

- Wait until they start sucking again, then give another gentle push on the plunger. Pause after another three to five seconds of drinking. Continue the feeding in this manner.

- Take a burping break about every five minutes. Your baby may or may not burp, but you'll want to give them the opportunity.

Remember that your baby is learning how to coordinate sucking, swallowing and breathing, and so you'll want to take these first feedings very slowly.

When a baby is learning to breastfeed/chestfeed, they have to suck for several seconds just to get a few drops of colostrum, and that's not an accident. The thick and sticky colostrum ensures the baby doesn't get overwhelmed or choke. Imitate nature as best you can, and stretch the finger feeding out to a minimum of 15 minutes. That's how long it takes the "I'm full signal" to reach your baby's brain (pg. 89).

By day three, when you're offering about an ounce of milk at every feeding, switching to a bottle makes sense. Ask the hospital for some ready-to-feed formula bottle nipples. These screw onto most colostrum cups nicely, creating a perfectly sized mini-bottle.

Pumping Plan for Day One and Two

- Hold your baby skin-to-skin before you pump. This raises your level of oxytocin, which helps milk flow. If holding your baby isn't possible, a quick, gentle breast/chest massage, and warming up the breasts/chest with a warm washcloth can also help milk flow.

- Start by hand expressing, about three to five minutes on each side.

- Then double pump for about 10 minutes. (Moms of twins will want to pump for 20 minutes.)

- If you are trying to establish a full milk supply, repeat every two to three hours during the day, and every three to four hours overnight, for a total of eight sessions every 24 hours.

- It's okay to give yourself up to a six-hour stretch of sleep, once a day. However, while trying to establish your supply, try not to go any longer than six hours without pumping. After about two weeks, when your milk supply is fairly set, you can experiment with stretching out your pumping sessions and possibly dropping some if you are producing more milk than you need.

As I've mentioned, for the first two or three days, it's normal to see only small amounts of colostrum. Around three days after birth, your breasts/chest should start to feel much fuller, warmer, and heavier. You may notice leaking in between pumping sessions and will start to collect more milk when you pump.

How Much Milk Does My Baby Need?

The volume guidelines in this chart are from The Academy of Breastfeeding Medicine.[13] Expect your baby to eat close to these amounts at least eight times every 24 hours. This is also about how much milk you should be expressing every time you pump, if you're pumping eight times every 24 hours.

Newborn Feeding Plan	
Day One	2–10 ml per feeding
Day Two	5–15 ml per feeding
Day Three	15–30 ml per feeding
Day Four	30–60 ml per feeding

The above is a rough guideline. When you practice responsive bottle feeding (Chapter Nine) with a healthy full-term baby, you'll be watching your baby's cues to know when they're still hungry and when they're full. This will help you give them the volume they need.

If you are not pumping the above amounts, or your baby is asking for more than what you have, supplement with formula, or if you're open to it, try nursing them until they are satisfied (a baby who is latched well does a great job at getting out any thick and sticky colostrum that the pump may have left behind). Keep following the pumping/hand expression plan, and you should see your supply gradually come up to meet the baby's demand.

After the fourth day of life, your baby's milk intake will continue to increase:

- Around the end of the first week, baby will be eating around 2 ounces per feeding, about eight times a day.

- Around the end of the second week, baby will be eating around 2–3 ounces per feeding, about eight times a day.

- This will gradually increase until the end of their first month, when they'll drink around 3–4 ounces per feeding, about eight times a day.

From one month old until six months old, most babies will drink around 3–4 ounces per feeding, about eight times a day. Some babies may take slightly larger volumes less frequently. The average daily intake of milk for a baby over four weeks old ranges from 24–32 ounces.[12,13] When a baby starts solids, their intake of milk may go down by a few ounces daily. You'll know you're feeding the "right" amount if your baby is putting out the diapers we expect to see, gaining weight on track, and giving you 2–3 hour stretches of satisfaction after most feedings (pg. 127).

Please Note: *All babies have different needs, and the above are just general recommendations. Talk to your pediatrician to make sure your baby is getting the right amount of milk.*

Pumping Plan for Day Three and Beyond

Once you feel your breasts filling and see more milk flowing, which usually happens around day three, try stopping the hand expression, and using only your pump.

- To call in a full milk supply, pump eight times every 24 hours.
- Double pump for 15 minutes each session. (25 minutes for parents with twins.)
- Try not to go longer than six hours between pumping sessions for the first two weeks.

Some parents become very engorged when their milk increases in volume. The pump can sometimes make engorgement worse by pulling swelling (it's not just milk filling your breasts/chest) down into your areola. The super swollen tissue can squeeze the milk ducts shut which restricts the milk flow. You'll know this is the case if you feel very full and try to pump… but little to nothing comes out!

If this happens to you, continue combining hand expression with pumping through the period of engorgement, which usually only lasts a day or two. Start with a few minutes of hand expression until things feel a little softer, and then try the pump. If your breasts are so swollen and firm that even hand expression is difficult, use a technique called "reverse pressure softening." Reverse pressure softening shifts the swelling out of your areola, temporarily softening the area so that you can hand express.

To use reverse pressure softening:
1. Place all four fingers and your thumb closely around your nipple, encircling it.
2. Firmly press into the swollen tissue.
3. Hold this pressure for one to three minutes. (The longer you hold it, the softer the areola will be when you release the hold.)
4. When you release your fingers, immediately start hand expressing.

Once you have released some milk, it's ok to try the pump. In between pumping sessions, place cold packs on your breasts/chest to help reduce the swelling and inflammation (heat tends to make it worse), and talk to your health care provider about taking ibuprofen, which also reduces inflammation. After the engorgement settles down, the pump should start working well on its own.

Reassess your plan after two weeks:

- Do you have the amount of milk that you want in a way that's working for you? Then keep your schedule as-is.
- Are you producing more than what your baby is eating? You might consider dropping a pumping session (pg. 125).
- Is your supply not meeting your baby's demand? It may be time to add some more pumping to your life, and be sure and read Chapter Six, "How Do I Boost My Supply?".

Once you have fine-tuned your plan, you can live in this flow state (pun intended) until about a week before you go back to work. At that time, I advise shifting your pumping schedule over to what it will look like during your workday. This gives your body time to adjust to the new routine, which may help prevent a dip in your supply after you return to work.

To wrap up this chapter, I want to remind you that just like with every aspect of baby feeding, there is no one "right way" to exclusively pump. There's only what works best for you, your baby, and your family. It's okay to change your plans, every feeding if necessary! As long as your baby is fed and loved, you're doing a great job.

Are you ready to talk bottles? Let's move on!

How Do I Exclusively Pump?

PART II:
The Plot Thickens with Bottle Feeding

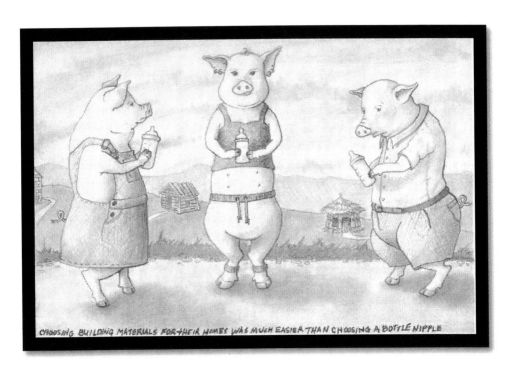

CHOOSING BUILDING MATERIALS FOR THEIR HOMES WAS MUCH EASIER THAN CHOOSING A BOTTLE NIPPLE

CHAPTER EIGHT:
DOES THE WAY
I BOTTLE FEED MATTER?

Before I teach the "how" of what I like to call "responsive bottle feeding" (a.k.a. "paced bottle feeding"), I want to share the WHY behind it. This will help you and your bottle-feeding helpers get on board with a bottle-feeding method that probably sounds very different than what you're used to.

To begin, let's consider how we drink and eat, as adults:

- Do we drink lying down?
- Do we drink in one continuous chugging session? (and I'm not talking about your college days.)
- Do we stop eating when we feel full, or when all the food is gone?

Most of us answered that we drink sitting up, take breaks, and stop eating when we're full. I know that last point gets a little tricky, as some of us were raised to be members of the "clean your plate" club, and sometimes on Thanksgiving we can be a little more, uh... *assertive* in our eating habits? But we all know it's best to stop eating when we feel full, and not when we need to unbutton our pants.

Now imagine a baby being bottle fed. What do you see in your mind's eye?

Most of us picture a caregiver holding the baby in a reclined position. The caregiver holds the bottle in the baby's mouth with the bottom of the bottle pointing up towards the ceiling. The baby chugs the bottle until the bottle is empty.

Babies are just mini-humans, and their little bodies operate in the same way ours do. This raises the question: Why are we asking our babies to eat/drink in a way that we don't?

You probably know the answer, which stems from an old wives' tale. It's a very spooky story, one that involves that evil villain AIR, that lurks in the bottle nipple, trying to maliciously connive its way into your baby's sensitive tummy and wreak havoc. We've come to believe that if there's ANY air in that bottle nipple, any at all—it will give the baby terrible gas and cause misery for all involved.

It makes sense on the surface that if we let a baby *drink* air, they'd blow up like a balloon. It also makes sense that to avoid this, we would need to hold the bottle as vertically as possible, and not allow air in the nipple.

But what if I told you that this old wives' tale is fixed firmly in the fantasy Fairy Tale World, and has no basis in our Dairy Tale reality? And that in fact, feeding a baby using this older, tradional bottle-feeding method may actually be *causing* the gas and fussing that we're trying to avoid in the first place?

Avoiding Air Intake

To think it through, I want you to imagine yourself in some situations that are similar to what a bottle-fed baby faces.

Scenario One: You're lying on your back, with your hands taped to your sides. Your friend puts a bottle of water into your mouth. Gravity causes the water to flow right away, so you have no choice but to start drinking. Or *chugging*, rather, as the water is flowing quite rapidly. How long can you chug like this before you need to stop and breathe? Five seconds? Ten? Unfortunately in this scenario, your friend doesn't offer you any breaks, and so you just have to grab a few breaths whenever you can, and pretty much continuously drink until the bottle is empty.

Scenario Two: Now imagine sitting upright, still without the use of your hands. Your friend taps the water bottle to your lips. You open your mouth to signal you're ready, and they insert the bottle in a more horizontal position. At this angle, the water flows more slowly so you're able to sip instead of chugging. Your friend lowers the bottle every few seconds to give you a break. When you're ready to drink again, you open your mouth, and they bring the bottle back up. And when you're all done, you stop opening your mouth and your friend takes the bottle away.

In which scenario would you be more likely to swallow air?

The first one, right?

In the second scenario, no one gets nervous about swallowing air, even though in both scenarios, air was getting into your mouth. Air always gets into our mouths when we drink, because we're not vacuum sealed to our cups. (Babies *are* actually vacuum sealed to the breast/chest, which is why they can lie down to drink there without any issues.) If you're skeptical about the idea of taking in air, take a sip of your beverage and pay attention to how you inhale a little before you start drinking. And notice how this doesn't cause any issues because when you're sitting up, you have space and time to swallow the liquid and breathe out the air.

In contrast, think about drinking with your head thrown all the way back, like when you chug a bottle of water after exercising. This is a similar situation to lying flat and drinking. When air gets into our mouths while we're chugging, we're not able to easily breathe it out, and so we swallow it. You know it's true because at the end of a chugging session, you tend to burp!

If you're following my line of thinking, you can see why the baby who lies flat and chugs is likely taking in more air than the baby who sits up and sips.

All of that being said, a baby swallowing a little air usually isn't a big problem. As long as the caregiver burps the baby every few minutes, any swallowed air comes right back up (sometimes with a little milk to keep things interesting) and life goes on (with more laundry). However, there are some babies who do get super uncomfortable after swallowing air, and for this baby, sitting upright to drink becomes especially important.

Traditional Bottle-Feeding Problems

Whether or not swallowed air causes issues for your baby, there are three other *bigger* problems that can occur when a baby lies flat and chugs their meal. Let's go through these issues one by one.

Traditional Bottle-Feeding Problem # 1: Overfeeding

I said earlier that babies' bodies work just like ours when it comes to drinking. And while that's *mostly* true, there is slight difference in that babies under 12 weeks old have a suck/swallow reflex. This means they have no voluntary control over their sucking and swallowing: When a hungry baby feels something touch the roof of their mouth (breast, bottle, pacifier or finger), their suck reflex is triggered. And if milk starts flowing, their swallow reflex is triggered.

These reflexes are important to keep in mind while bottle feeding because most bottles flow without the baby having to suck on the nipple. (Hold your bottle upside down and see if it drips.) When the caregiver holds the bottle vertically, the milk flows immediately, the baby's suck and swallow reflexes are triggered, and the rapid drinking begins. Due to their reflexes, the baby can't actually stop drinking until the bottle is empty. And that usually happens very quickly, which leads me to ask:

How long does it take you to know you're full?

Most people would answer "about 15–20 minutes." Once again, babies' bodies work similarly to ours, and so if the bottle feeding is finished in under 15 minutes, the baby may still look hungry, but only because their brain hasn't received the "I'm full" signal yet. The hungry-looking baby prompts the caregiver to make another bottle, and the baby chugs this one, too. By the time the baby's brain has received the "I'm full" signal from the stomach, it's likely they ate more than they needed.

I'm sure you've heard about how formula fed babies are more likely to be overweight than breastfed/chestfed babies.[21] An interesting question is how much of this issue is due to the formula itself and how much is due to the way in which these babies were bottle fed? Could we reduce the rates of overweight children just by slowing down the bottle feeds and paying closer attention to the baby's cues? There is little research in this area, but it makes sense that evidence point to "yes"[22,23] (and it definitely doesn't hurt anything to slow feedings down).

Overfeeding not only causes potential issues for the baby, but can also cause issues for the parents. If a baby is being overfed with pumped milk, you might start thinking you have a low supply since you can't keep up with your baby's demand. This is a common problem for babies who go to daycare. At the end of the day, the daycare staff tells the parent, "We ran out of milk, you need to pump more." If this happens to you, have a talk with them about how quickly your baby is drinking the milk before you assume your supply is the issue. As a reminder, a typical meal for babies over the age of one month is 3–4 ounces of milk per bottle.

Traditional Bottle-Feeding Problem # 2: Bottle Refusal

I get calls from parents when their baby is around 8–12 weeks old, and they say something like:

"He'd been taking the bottle fine for weeks, but then one day just started refusing. I have to go back to work and really need him to take the bottle!"

This is a baby who was seemingly taking the bottle "fine" but in reality, was likely getting stressed by the fast flow. This baby sucked and swallowed the milk due to their reflexes being triggered; there was no other choice. But once the baby began to lose these reflexes (somewhere around 12 weeks old), they were finally able to tell their caregiver, "I don't like being fed this way," by refusing the bottle.

I advise these parents to reintroduce the bottle in a kind, gentle and fun way. This can take time to resolve, and as you can imagine, can be quite stressful if the parent has to go back to work before the baby is consistently taking the bottle.

Traditional Bottle-Feeding Problem #3: Breast/Chest Refusal

On the opposite end of the spectrum are babies who start refusing the breast/chest due to the rapid bottle feeds. I hear from these parents a short time after the bottle was introduced:

"She was breastfeeding fine, but now she just screams and will only take the bottle, what can I do?"

Unlike the baby in the example above, this baby figured out how to chug their bottle down without much stress, and then started to actually *prefer* that quick flow. When brought to the breast/chest, they get upset that they have to work and be patient. You may have heard of this problem being referred to as "nipple confusion." However, this baby isn't "confused" at all, but rather showing a clear preference for the fast flow of the bottle.

I advise parents in this situation to try and "level the playing field" by slowing down the flow of the bottle and speeding up the flow at the breast/chest. This plan involves time, energy, and patience...and usually some level of frustration.

Luckily, you can largely avoid all of these bottle-feeding problems by introducing the bottle around three weeks postpartum and practicing "responsive bottle feeding," which you'll learn in the next chapter.

One last thing we need before we start bottle feeding...a bottle! Let's talk through how to choose a bottle that will up your odds of success switching back and forth between bottle and boob.

How Do I Choose a Bottle?

You're in the baby store, standing in front of a wall of bottles. You really had no idea there were this many to choose from and feel overwhelmed. You pick up a bottle, and the package announces, "more like the breast than ever!" And you think, "Yes, this bottle nipple DOES look like a breast!" The base of this bottle nipple is wide, and it has a nipple sticking up out of the center. It makes sense that a bottle that looks like a breast would be better for a breastfeeding/chestfeeding baby, but I'm here to help you understand why in most cases, this probably isn't true.

While the wider-based bottle nipples indeed resemble a breast *at rest*, they don't look anything like a breast *inside of a nursing baby's mouth*, which is what we're actually shooting for. When your baby latches deeply, they stretch your breast/chest tissue far up into the roof of their mouth and your nipple becomes elongated as they suck. Therefore, it is a longer, thinner bottle nipple—or one that moves very gradually from thinner to wider—that best imitates this situation. There are several bottle brands that make nipples like this, and I'd encourage you to try out a few before deciding which is the "best" one for you and your baby.

The potential problem with the traditional wider-based nipples is that it's easy for a baby to slip off of the base and end up sucking on the bottle nipple like a straw. These babies have the potential to get back on the breast/chest and try to suck their parent's nipple like a straw (ouch!).

What if you happen to already be using a wide-based nipple, and your baby is doing great switching back and forth? As the old saying goes, "If it ain't broke, don't fix it." Many babies do just fine on any bottle nipple you give them, and if you have one of these easy-peasy babies—you don't need to change a thing. Starting out with a longer thinner nipple is just general advice to up the odds of success for parents who haven't bought bottles yet, or who are having issues with the wide-based nipples.

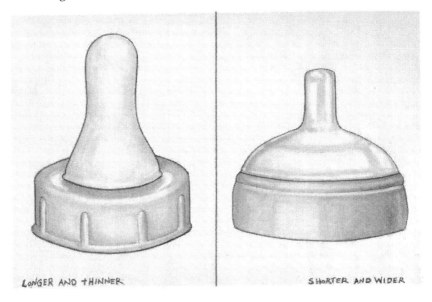

LONGER AND THINNER   SHORTER AND WIDER

Whichever bottle you end up buying, make sure the nipple is "slow flow." This is to help make sure baby doesn't get too much milk too quickly, which may lead to overfeeding and an upset tummy. You might not ever need a faster-flowing nipple, as most babies do well staying on the slow flow for as long as they take a bottle.

However, I occasionally encourage parents to go up a flow speed if:

- The bottle feed regularly takes longer than 30 minutes.
- The baby sucks so hard that the nipple collapses.
- The baby starts popping on and off the nipple.
- The baby falls asleep early in the feeding due to the slow flow.
- The baby gets frustrated with the flow speed and fusses or cries during the feeding.

Therefore, if there's a reason to size up the flow speed, go for it. But don't feel like you *have* to, just because the bottle manufacturer said so. Having you buy new nipples every three months is great for their bottom line, but not necessarily great for your bottle feeding routine.

An interesting fact about the bottle industry is that no one regulates or monitors the designation "slow flow." This means every brand of "slow flow" nipple flows at a different rate. I've even seen different nipples of the same brand, all categorized as "slow flow"—flow differently! (You can test this at home by filling your bottle nipples with water and comparing their drip rate when help upside-down.)

All of this is just to put a point on the fact that there's no one "right" nipple for every baby, and that watching your baby's behavior closely during the bottle feeding is the best way to figure out their ideal nipple flow speed.

Okay, you have your milk, you have your bottle, and you're ready to give it to your baby. Let the next chapter be your guide to better bottle feeding

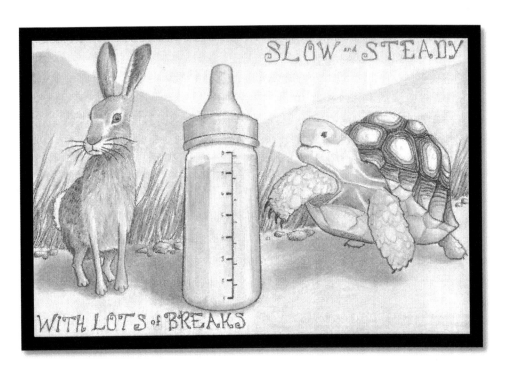

CHAPTER NINE:

How do I Introduce the Bottle?

When you're really hungry, I'll bet you're not in the mood to learn a new skill— and neither is your baby. Babies suck and swallow differently on the bottle than they do on the breast, and so there is a learning curve when you introduce the bottle. Some babies find this an easy transition, while others need a little more time to become efficient bottle feeders. To up the chances of success, try introducing the bottle when baby is awake, alert, in a good mood, and just a *little* hungry.

Before You Get Started

Wash and sterilize your bottle parts before using them. Follow the bottle manufacturer's instructions and talk to your pediatrician to see how often you need to sterilize your baby's bottle parts.

Only put about an ounce of milk in the first bottle you offer. Once your baby's lips touch the bottle nipple, bacteria are introduced into the milk and it needs to be used within two hours (one hour if it's a formula bottle) or thrown away.[8] In the unlikely event your baby refuses the bottle, throwing away an ounce of milk will be much less heartbreaking than throwing away three ounces or more.

Responsive Bottle Feeding, Step-by-Step

1. Hold baby upright and touch the bottle nipple to their lips. A hungry baby will open their mouth.

   If the baby doesn't open, do not force the nipple in, as this can lead to bottle refusal over time. Stop and try again later.

2. Place the nipple in their mouth and help them latch deeply. Whichever kind of bottle nipple you're using, make sure the baby's mouth is opened widely, and their lips are flanged outwards, like a fish. The baby will start to suck and swallow.

3. Keep the bottle as horizontal as possible, which helps slow the flow of milk. There may be some air in the nipple, which you'll recall from the last chapter is totally fine.

4. Watch your baby carefully. Depending on how quickly the bottle is flowing, they may be able to take breaks on their own. If you see your baby stop sucking, tilt the bottle down so that the nipple stays in their mouth, but no milk is flowing.

   Also watch your baby for signs that they are overwhelmed.

   An overwhelmed baby might:

   - Squinch their eyebrows in a "worried look."
   - Open their eyes very widely.
   - Become rigid and arch their back.
   - Put out their hands out in a "stop" position.
   - Dribble milk out of their mouth.
   - Cough and sputter.

   If you notice any of these behaviors, give the baby a break.

5. If the baby doesn't take a break, it's because they *can't* due to the rapid flow of milk. Help them "put down their dinner fork" by lowering the bottle about every three to five seconds. It's normal for the baby to keep sucking on the empty nipple for a second or two, but once they realize there's no milk flowing, they'll stop sucking and pause. When ready to drink, they'll start sucking again. That's your cue to tip the bottle back up and let milk flow.

    If despite my reassurances you (or more likely your parents or in-laws) are still worried about a baby sucking on an empty bottle nipple, there is another option to give the baby a break: Gently twist the bottle to break the suction, remove the nipple from your baby's mouth, and let it rest on their cheek. This will let the baby know that you're giving them a break, but not taking their food away. If they're still hungry after pausing, they'll turn back towards the nipple with an open mouth. This is your signal to continue the feeding.

6. Take a burping break every five minutes or so.

7. As the feeding goes on, the baby will take longer and longer pauses and eventually they'll fall asleep, turn their head away, and/or stop sucking. This means the baby is finished. Remember that the bottle feeding should take at least 15 minutes, so that the baby's brain has time to receive the "I'm full" signal from the stomach.

Please Note: *There may or may not be milk left in the bottle when the baby is done, but please throw it away instead of trying to get the baby to drink it. I've seen caregivers twist the bottle in the baby's mouth to make them finish every drop of milk. Twisting the nipple causes the milk to flow, and then the baby's swallow reflex forces them to drink it. This is a forced feeding situation, and I want you to think about someone demanding you keep eating after you've told them "I'm full." (If you happen to be a member of the "clean your plate" club, you actually know exactly how this feels.) In addition to overfeeding the baby, this forced feeding may lead to future bottle refusal.*

Also Note: *Once your baby is around 12 weeks old, they start to gain voluntary control over their suck/swallow reflexes and become better at pacing themselves.*

Trouble Stretching the Feeding Out to 15 Minutes?

Even when using responsive bottle feeding, you may still end up with a bottle feeding that clocks in under 15 minutes.

In cases like these, a pacifier can help. When a hungry baby goes to the breast/chest, they are not instantly gratified the way they are when they start a bottle feeding. They need to suck for at least a few seconds at the breast before the milk starts to flow, and then the milk naturally ebbs and flows throughout the feeding. To make the bottle feeding better imitate this natural pattern, give your baby the pacifier for about 30 seconds before starting the bottle feed, and then use it intermittently throughout the feeding. Every few minutes, stop the feeding, burp your baby, and then give them the pacifier for 30–60 seconds before bringing the bottle back. As well as spreading out the length of the feeding, using the pacifier also teaches your baby that they'll still need to do some work while bottle feeding, which helps lower the risk of breast refusal.

Did your first bottle feeding go well?

Congrats!

How to Incorporate Bottle Feeding into Your Life

You now have a baby who can both breastfeed/chestfeed and bottle feed, which means you can enlist helpers for feedings. Offer at least a few bottles a week, to keep your baby used to switching back and forth.

Here's a few ways you can keep the bottle in rotation:

- Offer ½ ounce to 1 ounce of milk after nursing in the evening, before bedtime.
- Offer a full bottle (3–4 ounces) in the afternoon to replace a breast-feed/chestfeed (pump at the same time to maintain your supply and stash this milk in your freezer).
- Offer an ounce of milk during a cluster-feeding stretch.
- Offer a full bottle to replace a middle-of-the-night nursing session (more on this in a bit).
- Pump and bottle feed to replace any breastfeeding/chestfeeding, for any reason (e.g. you want a break!).

As you can see, there is no one "right way" to combine breastfeeding/chest-feeding and bottle feeding. Do what works for you! However, there are a few things to keep in mind:

- Make sure you offer the bottle at least a few times a week. (I've met babies who started refusing the bottle after taking just one week off.)
- To keep a full milk supply, you'll need to pump for any 3–4 ounce bottle that you give (pumped milk or formula), somewhere in your 24-hour day (i.e. you don't need to pump at the same time your baby is getting the bottle.)
- You can choose to use small amounts of formula for bottle feeding practice. This won't impact your supply as long as you are only using about an ounce of formula once a day or every other day and getting in at least eight good breast stimulations every 24 hours.
- If your *plan* is to combine formula with breastfeeding/chestfeeding, then you don't need to worry about pumping. Your supply will naturally drop at those times of the day when you are regularly using formula.

Middle-of-the-Night Bottles

Many nursing parents have their partner take over a nightshift feeding with the bottle. You may be wondering if your supply will drop if you don't get up and pump while your baby eats. And the answer is yes, your supply WILL drop, but only during that particular stretch of the night. (Which is exactly what you want!)

Remember that your milk supply is based on demand. If you pump while baby is getting a bottle at 2 a.m., you've just swapped out feeding your baby for feeding Pumpy. Pumping at 2 a.m. tells your body, "Keep making milk at 2 a.m., the robot baby wants it." And your body will do as it's asked.

But the whole point of the overnight bottle was for you to get more sleep, right?

By keeping a full breast/chest at 2 a.m., you'll be sending the message to your body, "Stop making milk at 2 a.m., no one wants it." And your body will do as it's asked. However, it *will* take a few nights of feeling full to make the 2 a.m. milk supply go down. This means that the first night your baby gets a 2 a.m. bottle, your full boobs will probably wake you up, saying, "hey, you're supposed to be feeding a baby!" When this happens, take a little bit of milk out, just enough to be able to go back to sleep. After a few days of feeling comfortably full at 2 a.m., your supply will gradually decrease, and you'll be able to start sleeping through that stretch of the night.

There's really no need to stress about this nighttime milk going away. As long as you're pumping once a day, you're essentially just shifting milk from the nighttime over to the daytime, which means your overall supply stays the same.

You are now a pumping and bottle-feeding parent and can start thinking through the logistics of returning to work. In the next few chapters, I'll help you with a plan to make this as easy as possible

Part III:
They Lived Happily Ever After Going Back to Work

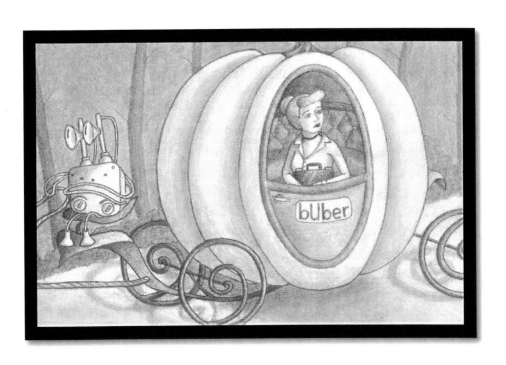

CHAPTER TEN:
Back-to-Work:
The Practical

You're reading this book because pumping at work is probably something you'd like to do, but I want you to know that it's your *legal right*, as well. Type "break time for nursing mothers," into your search engine, and you will find the Department of Labor's website,[24] which explains your federal right to pump. Tack your state onto the end of the above search phrase (e.g. "break time for nursing mothers Texas") to see what's up in your neck of the woods.

Pumping and the Law

You can read the entire law for yourself, but here's the gist of it: Most employers (small business owners have some exemptions) are required to provide break time and a space to pump for up to one year after birth. The space provided must be private and cannot be a bathroom.

Now that you know you *can* pump at work, let's talk logistics.

Items to Keep at Work

If you are able to store items at work, bring the following things in a few days before you start back. This way you'll have less to pack in general and your first day won't be overly hectic. If keeping items at work isn't an option, keep them in your pumping bag or car.

Items to Keep at Work

- An extra pumping kit (tubes, valves, or anything that could break.)

- Spare batteries if your pump takes them.

- A spare pumping bra.

- Breast pads. If you get that tingly feeling like a letdown is about to happen, cross your arms across your chest and put pressure on your nipples. This works well to minimize leaks. The breast pads will catch the rest.

- An extra shirt or two for when the above fails. FYI - milk spots are less visible on prints.

- A "Do Not Disturb" sign for the pumping room door.

- Snacks and drinks. Eating well and staying hydrated help maintain your milk supply.

- Extra milk storage bags and bottles.

- Pictures of your baby.

When you go in to drop off your things, consider bringing your baby with you. Meeting your baby can help your colleagues connect your upcoming pumping breaks with a real live (adorable) little human and foster general goodwill around pumping.

Items to Keep in Your Pumping Bag

- Your pump, all pump parts, and power cord.

- Pumping bra.

- Bottles.

- A hand pump for if you get stuck in traffic, the power goes out, your pump breaks, etc.

- Masking tape and markers for recording the date.

- Surface wipes and pump wipes.

- Hand sanitizer.

- A spare phone charger, in case you run out of juice while pumping.

- They probably don't fit in your bag, but don't forget your insulated cooler bag and cold packs.

- Consider keeping a checklist in your bag and run through it every time you pack.

Please note: *You may have heard that mothers with healthy babies over three months old refrigerate their pump parts in a large zip-top bag and wash them after every other use. CDC guidance states, "As soon as possible after pumping, clean pump parts," but doesn't specify a time limit.[3] If conditions at your job make it difficult (or gross) to wash pump parts, talk to your pediatrician to see if this fridge hack might work for you.*

One Week Before You Go Back

- Start pumping on your new schedule. For example, if you'll be pumping at work at 9, 12, and 3, do this at home, and give your baby a bottle instead of nursing them. This gives your body and your baby time to adjust to the new normal.

- Consider starting your baby at daycare a day or two before you go back. This trial run can give you an idea of the flow of your new schedule and allow you to tweak it as needed. As a bonus, you can go out to lunch, go visit a friend, or even just take a nap.

- Visit your workplace to drop off pumping supplies, have everyone meet your baby, and scope out the state of the pumping room and fridge.

- Sort out any pumping room scheduling issues.

Your First Week Back

- Plan to return on a Thursday, so that you only need to work two days before taking a break.

- Schedule your pumping breaks on your shared calendar, and honor your body and your baby by sticking to them.

- Keep a running list of things you need to bring, or tweaks you need to make. If you don't write it down, you'll probably forget.

- Pack your pumping and diaper bags the night before, to make your mornings as calm as possible.

- Identify your allies. Check in with anyone else who has a new baby or had one recently.

- Go outside when you can, and take in some fresh air and sunshine.

- Don't forget to eat and drink, as this impacts your milk supply.

- Remember that getting back into the swing of things at work will take time. Treat yourself gently and give yourself lots of grace.

What if I Work from Home?

If you work from home and your baby is home with you, you may have the option of breastfeeding/chestfeeding instead of pumping. This option largely depends on how flexible your schedule is and how predictable your baby is. Some moms who work from home play it by ear and make their decisions feeding by feeding. If they're about to pump, they check to see if the baby is hungry, and if things line up, they breastfeed/chestfeed. If baby is hungry but mom is in the middle of a meeting, baby gets a bottle and mom pumps later. Whatever works!

Now that you know the practical side of being a pumping parent, let's talk about the mental and emotional side of things. Read on to help you return to work gracefully and with a positive mental attitude.

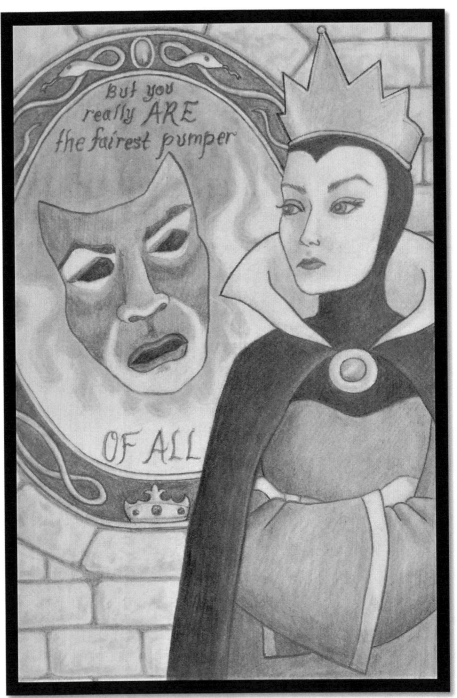

CHAPTER ELEVEN:
Back-to-Work:
The Emotional

You've gotten your pumping routine down, your baby is taking the bottle like a champ, and your pumping bag is packed. Great job! Before you rush back into working life, let's spend a few minutes reflecting on your feelings. Are you excited? Anxious? Relieved?

It's normal to feel a variety of emotions as you get ready for this next chapter in your life. Being pregnant, giving birth, caring for a newborn, and moving back into working life are all big shifts, and it's helpful to acknowledge and process the emotions that come along with these changes.

Back-to-Work Guilt

One feeling that pops up for many parents during this time is guilt.

Just like with other forms of parenting guilt, when it comes to going back to work, it may feel like you're damned if you do, and you're damned if you don't.

Some parents feel guilty about leaving their babies when they go back to work. Others look forward to going back to work and so feel guilty for NOT feeling guilty about leaving their babies.

It seems that just about every parent is feeling guilty for one reason or another. Where does all of this guilt leave us? And how can we banish it once and for all?

The way I see it, there are two types of guilt—helpful and unhelpful.

Helpful guilt is an emotion that arises after one has done something illegal, immoral, or unethical. For example: If a person took something that didn't belong to them, they might feel guilty afterwards. In this case, guilt is potentially a helpful emotion, as it might prompt the person to return the stolen item, apologize, and change their ways. To put it in other words, helpful guilt is capable of prompting positive change.

Guilt as it relates to going back to work is always unhelpful. It occurs in a situation where the parent has done nothing wrong and it only brings negative changes—there is nothing positive to be gained from unhelpful guilt. There is often non-rational, negative self-talk happening that impacts a parent's ability to function, both at home and at work. What's worse, a parent in the throes of back-to-work guilt often has trouble enjoying themselves or their baby…which means this unhelpful guilt really needs to go.

If you have been living with guilt, try using the following techniques to move into a kinder, more reality-based state of mind.

Banishing Guilt

Take a few deep breaths and imagine you're breathing in white light. Let the light fill your whole body. Hold it for a few seconds, and then exhale. As you breathe out, visualize the guilt, anxiety and stress leaving you in a cloud of gray smoke. Inhale white light and exhale gray smoke at least three times, but take as much time as you need to feel more relaxed. When you're ready, say the following affirmations to yourself.

Guilt Around Returning to Work

If you have been feeling guilty about being apart from your baby, affirm:

- "I am working to create a wonderful life for myself and my child."

- "My baby is in the best care possible."

- "Our caregiver makes my baby's happiness their top priority."

- "I am giving my baby the opportunity to trust other caregivers and socialize with other children."

- "I intentionally reconnect with my baby at the end of every day and treasure our time together more than ever."

Reflect on these affirmations daily, until you feel you no longer need them.

It's common for parents to struggle with the adjustment of being apart from their baby, and those first few days and weeks are often the hardest. I encourage you to give yourself at least a few months to adjust before making any decisions about leaving your job.

Guilt Around Wanting to Return to Work

If you have been feeling guilty about wanting to go back to work, affirm:

- "It is normal and healthy to spend time apart from my baby."

- "Taking time for myself makes me a better parent."

- "Being a parent is only one part of my identity."

- "I balance my needs with my family's needs."

- "I work so that I can provide a wonderful life for myself and my child."

Reflect on these affirmations daily, until you feel you no longer need them.

Understand that how you feel now, before returning to work, may change over time. You may dread going back to work and find you love it, or you may want to go back to work and then struggle. As you can't predict how you will feel, it's best to not worry about the future, take each day as it comes, and try not to judge yourself.

Regardless of whether you want to be at work or not, pumping at work is not usually something *anyone* looks forward to. To help this situation, try the following tips to make pumping as pleasant as possible. The more pleasant your pumping experience, the more pleasant your overall day. And the more pleasant your day, the more easily your milk can flow.

Tips for Making Pumping More Pleasant

- Buy a pumping bag you absolutely LOVE. This will make pumping a little more pleasant than a bag you're indifferent to (or worse, a bag you hate).

- For similar reasons, invest in a pumping bra and nursing clothes that you absolutely adore and feel fabulous in.

- Consider decorating your pump with stickers, rhinestones, and affirmations. This may seem silly, but looking at a pump that makes you smile is a plus for your mood.

- Write notes on your freezer storage bags about what your baby is up to. When you pull the milk out of the freezer weeks or months later, you can take a sweet trip down memory lane.

- Make friends with someone at work who is currently pumping or who has recently. Find ways to brighten each other's days.

- Don't apologize for having to pump, leaving to pick up your baby, calling out if your baby is sick, etc. This implies to others (and yourself!) that you are doing something wrong. Replace an apology with a "thank you." For example: Instead of saying, "I'm sorry, but I have to go pick up my baby now," try, "I need to jump out of this meeting to go pick up my baby, thank you for understanding."

- Consider a daycare provider who has a live video stream, or who sends you pics during the day. These visuals can set you at ease, which can make your pumping time more relaxing and rewarding.

Tips if You Notice a Dip

- Don't panic. Many parents experience a dip in their milk supply due to the stress of the transition. As the parent adjusts and the stress levels go down, the milk supply tends to go back to normal.

- Consider what *else* has changed. Commonly this supply dip is due to stress, however, there may be other factors at play. Many parents inadvertently drop a feeding/pumping session due to the overall schedule change, which would also cause a dip. Adding the missed breast/chest stimulation back in should bring the supply back up.

- Remember that breastfeeding/chestfeeding never has to be all-or-nothing. Many mothers use a temporary formula supplement, and some find a balance using both pumped milk and formula for the long haul.

- Keep the pump running for the entire 15–minute pumping session, even when no milk is flowing. This stimulation is boosting milk making hormones and "placing an order" for more milk.

- Switch your pump into fast/impatient baby mode whenever little to no milk is flowing. (pg. 22).

- Stay as relaxed as possible. Take deep breaths, turn off any negative voices in your head and replace them with positive thoughts. If you're not already, use the pumping affirmation on page 70.

- If you've been working during your pumping breaks, consider stopping if you can. Sometimes taking a TRUE break from work is necessary to get your body into a more relaxed state.

- Double check your pump parts. Have you replaced pump parts per the manufacturer's instructions?

- Double check your flange fit. Some parents need to go up a size after they've been pumping for a few weeks.

- Try not to stare at your pump bottles while pumping. Watch a funny video, read a magazine, or close your eyes and visualize rivers of milk. Some parents put socks over the bottles to break this habit.

- Are you eating, drinking and sleeping well? (And this includes eating and drinking at work!) If not, do what you can to get into a better routine.

- Up the amount of breastfeeding/chestfeeding/pumping you're doing at home, as this will help boost overall supply.

- Hold your baby skin-to-skin at home whenever you can. Your baby's skin against yours boosts your levels of oxytocin which helps more milk to flow.

- Are you using "hands-on" pumping? (pg. 65)

- Is pumping during your commute an option? To do this safely, you'll need to get setup and turn your pump on before you start driving and turn it off only once you are parked. NEVER EVER MESS WITH YOUR PUMP WHILE DRIVING. Some mothers find that larger bottles will rest on their legs, which helps them feel less nervous about milk overflowing the bottles or accidental spills. A towel on your lap is bonus spill security. Wearable pumps are terrific for pumping while commuting, but many moms use a standard pump and just wear a nursing cover.

- Re-read Chapter Six (pg. 57) for tips on boosting supply in general, and work with your health care provider and a lactation consultant to see if a milk-boosting supplement might be helpful in your case.

If you are a working parent who travels, the next chapter is for you.

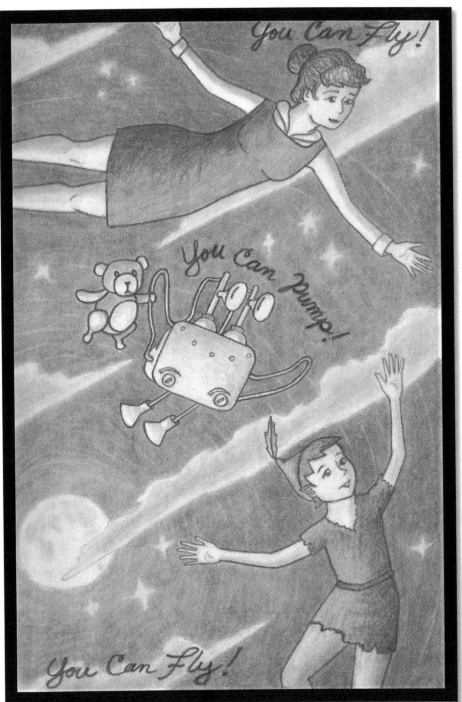

CHAPTER TWELVE:

How Do I Pump While Traveling?

Even though you'll be leaving parenting behind for a few days when you travel, sadly, you can't leave behind your pump. Pumpy will be subbing in for your baby full time during your travels, to maintain your supply and help you avoid plugged ducts.

Notice I didn't say Pumpy's job is to help you bring home as much pumped milk as possible? I want you to think about how much milk you really NEED to bring home, as your answer will hugely impact your travels.

Options for Saving Milk

Option One: Don't bring home ANY milk. Practically speaking, this is your easiest option. Many moms with a decent milk supply (pumping 3–5 ounces in place of breastfeeds) will be able to "pump and dump" while away, and then just go back to their usual routine when they get back home.

In this scenario, you don't need to pack a cooler and ice blocks. You don't need to secure multiple fridges. You don't need to talk to the TSA about the extra liquids you're carrying.

Sounds wonderful, but this plan doesn't come without its own challenge, which will be dumping every ounce of milk you pump down the drain. (I bet you cringed just now merely *thinking* about that.) But if you really don't NEED to bring it home, I'd encourage you to put on a brave face, pump and dump your milk, and enjoy your travels more freely.

Option Two: Bring home SOME milk. This option is for you if you have a borderline milk supply, you really don't want to use formula, and your freezer stash is going to take a major hit while you're away. In this case, choose a cooler bag to hold the amount of milk you're comfortable transporting. Then decide when you'll feel okay to pump and dump (maybe the milk you'll pump in the airport) and when you'll want to pump and store (maybe the milk you'll pump in your hotel room). You might also consider shipping home some pumped milk, to travel a little lighter.

Option Three: Bring home MOST of your milk. Some of you will want to bring home as much milk as possible for any number of reasons, and while tricky, it's totally possible with solid planning.

I didn't call this bullet "bring home ALL of your milk," because pumping in strange places (airplane bathrooms, for instance) lends itself to mishaps, shenanigans, and spills (and a few good stories to be sure.) If you expect to lose a little along the way, you'll feel a little less devastated when it happens.

If you are going to have more milk than what will fit into your cooler bags, or you don't want to be weighed down while traveling, you can ship some.

Type "shipping breast milk" into your search engine, and you'll find companies who specialize in this task (expensive but easier), as well as DIY instructions (cheaper but more involved). If you have a few extra bucks, going with a company who will make life easier is a strong move.

Now that you've decided how much milk you're bringing home, let's talk about life on the road with Pumpy.

What Will Your Travel Pumping Schedule Look Like?

You're probably wondering if you'll need to stay on the same schedule that you've become used to. And the answer, like so many things in life is, "it depends."

If you're going away for less than a week, and you're happy with your current baby feeding situation and milk supply, it makes sense to keep your schedule as close to normal as possible (you'll need to factor in any time zone changes).

If you're going away for longer, or you'd just prefer to be pumping less often while you're traveling, you can plan ahead and start cutting down before you leave (pg. 125). It's important that you don't just suddenly change your pumping schedule the day of departure, as this ups your chances of engorgement, leaking, plugged ducts and mastitis. If you give your body time to adjust before you leave, you'll be in good shape while on the road.

Keep in mind that if you do cut back on pumping while away, your supply will gradually drop. And it will take about a week of increased pumping/breastfeeding/chestfeeding once you're back home to get it back to normal. Depending on your freezer stash, this may mean you'll need to use some formula to keep your baby fed while your supply is lower than usual. But in the next section, I'm going to make a case for you to feel okay using some formula regardless of your travel pumping plan.

Backup, Plan "F"

You've probably heard the horror stories of freezer stashes needing to be tossed after the power went out or a chest freezer was accidentally unplugged, as well as stories of babies who just straight up refused to drink the frozen milk (pg. 37). I've also heard stories where the caregiver misunderstood how much milk to give at every feeding and used up the freezer stash too quickly. Imagine you are traveling and something like this happens. It's unlikely, but definitely possible in our less-than-perfect Dairy Tale World.

If you are having intense anxiety around the "what-ifs" connected to baby feeding while you're away, think about offering your baby a bottle of formula a few days before you leave. Chances are your baby will take it without a problem, and then you would just keep some formula in rotation so they stayed used to it (an ounce or two every other day is plenty). This would give you the peace of mind that your baby will be fed while you're away, no matter what. Plan "F" is not for every parent out there, but I want you to at least consider it, especially if you will be gone for more than a few days. Talk to your pediatrician if your baby has never had formula, as they can help you choose the right one (and maybe give you a free sample!).

Planning Ahead

It's a great idea to plan out when and where you'll be pumping, and where you'll be storing the pumped milk. To stay organized, keep all of your pumping-related details in a separate notebook. Below are a few things you'll want to jot down in your pumping planner:

- A pumping schedule for your travel days.

- A pumping schedule for your non-travel days.

- Where you're going to pump in the airport, hotel, workspace, etc. (Check out the Mamava app to help you locate their "lactation pods," found in many airports.)

- Contact info for managers at your hotels and workspaces. Let them know you will be pumping in advance of your arrival, and that you'll need a fridge.

- Print out your airline's pumped milk policies and get familiar with them. They may come in handy if you find yourself talking to an ignorant staff member.

You now have your pumping plan in place and are ready to pack. So…whatcha bringing?

Packing

No doubt about it, now that you're a pumping parent, you're going to have way more crap than usual when you fly.

An important consideration is whether you need to carry on your double electric pump. If your travel time from door to door is six hours or less, consider stashing your double electric pump in your checked bag and using your manual pump as needed.

Whether or not you decide to carry on your double electric pump, pack your pump parts in zip-top bags. This creates a barrier between grimy TSA fingers and your pump.

What to Pack in Your Carry-On Bags:

- Hand pump. Even if you have a super short flight and you are pump-ing on either end, bring your hand pump anyway. Getting delayed on the tarmac is bad. Hand expressing engorged breasts into the air-plane sink is much, much worse.

- Nursing cover.

- Breast pads.

- Extra shirt.

- Cooler pack (if you're not pumping and dumping).

- Hand and surface sanitizing wipes.

- Pump wipes. Buy a bottle of water once past security to rinse your pump parts, but pump wipes are good in a pinch.

- Snacks! (And be sure and stay hydrated during your flight, too.)

What to Pack in Your Checked Bag:

- Double Electric Pump (if you're not bringing it on the plane).
  - o Pump parts, plug, batteries, bottles and storage bags.
  - o Backup membranes and valves.
  - o Do you need an adapter for international travel? Bring a spare, as these are easily left behind while out and about.

- A cooler pack and cold blocks, if you're not bringing them on the plane. (Just don't forget them if you're planning to transport milk!)

- Extra milk storage bags.

- Extra zip-top bags for pump parts. (Are you going to refrigerate your flanges between sessions? Bring more than you think you'll use.)

- Extra shirts.

- Extra breast pads.

And those are my tips for traveling parents!

CONCLUSION:
GO FORTH AND PUMP

While pumping is not anyone's idea of a fairy tale, it doesn't have to be a horror story. Learning how to overcome pumping obstacles to gain comfort, confidence and balance is truly a hero's journey, and I hope this book has placed you firmly on that path.

Even after reading this book, you may still feel overwhelmed. This is normal, as it's definitely a lot to take in. Just like there was a learning curve with breastfeeding/chestfeeding and newborn care, there will be a learning curve with pumping. Take things one day at a time and give yourself tons of grace while you practice putting your new knowledge into action.

You CAN do this!

If things are not going as expected, always get help before you give up, and remember that however you are feeding your baby, you're doing a great job.

You are ready. I believe in you, am proud of you, and know you're going to rock the world of Dairy Tales.

Happy pumping!

Appendix A:
WEANING

When you are ready to cut back on breastfeeding/chestfeeding/pumping, or stop altogether, you'll find a gradual weaning plan is a good way to stay comfortable and lower your risk of plugged ducts and mastitis.

General Weaning Plan

- Choose the breastfeeding/chestfeeding/pumping session you enjoy the least and drop it.

- Spread out your remaining feeding/pumping sessions in a way that makes sense.

- If you feel uncomfortably full during or after the skipped session, pump or hand express just a little to get comfortable, but stay fairly full. A full breast is the only way to tell your body to "make less milk."

- After 3–5 days, when your body has had time to adjust and you're not feeling overly full anymore, go ahead and cut the next session.

- While you are dropping breastfeeding/chestfeeding sessions, continue to spend lots of snuggle time with your baby. This helps them with the adjustment, so they don't feel like they are losing their physical connection with you.

- If you do the math, you'll realize a gradual weaning plan can take weeks to complete. Plan accordingly if you are trying to totally dry up before returning to work.

APPENDIX B:
HOW TO KNOW BABY IS GETTING ENOUGH

Excerpt from "Breastfeeding 101: Prepare for the Suck"

There are three good ways to know that your baby is getting enough milk:

1. **Count your baby's diapers**. One wet and one poop diaper on day one. Two and two on day two. Three and three on day three. Four and four on day four. On day five and beyond, you will want to see six or more wet diapers and three poops every 24 hours (poops need to be the size of a quarter or larger to count).

   Also pay attention to the color and texture changes of the poops. They will start out black and sticky on day one and two, turn greenish and thin out a little around day three and then become yellow and seedy with a more watery-mustardy texture by day five. If your diapers are adding up and changing color as expected, your baby is getting enough milk.

2. **Watch your baby's behavior.** Does baby show hunger cues before feeding, wide rhythmic sucking during a feeding, and then look satisfied and relaxed at the end? Are they giving you at least a couple of two or three hour stretches of happy and relaxed (or sleeping) behavior? If you've answered "yes," these are great signs that baby is getting enough.

3. **Monitor your baby's weight.** Most babies lose weight in the first few days of life. This is normal and expected as they are not eating large amounts yet. A 5–7% weight loss is considered normal. Anything greater than this and you should get some help. Once your milk increases in volume around day three, your baby should start gaining about 2/3 of an ounce to 1 ounce every day. Your pediatrician will help you keep track. If your baby's weight gain is on target, you're doing great.

If any of the above seem off, your baby might **not** be getting enough milk. If you are not getting the diapers you should, if baby is crying and showing hunger cues around the clock despite frequent feeds, if they aren't gaining weight well, or if you feel like something is just not right, then it's time to get help. Call your pediatrician, and then contact a lactation consultant to trouble shoot and come up with a feeding plan.

APPENDIX C:
ᚠAINᖴUᒪ ᑭUᗰᑭINᏀ

If you are experiencing pain with pumping, know that this is not normal and something needs to change. Review the checklist below to see what might be causing you distress.

- Are your flanges the right size?
  - ○ If your nipples are rubbing up against the inside of the tunnel of the flange, your flanges are too small.
    - ▪ **Please Note:** *There are some lactation consultants who will tell you your nipples should rub the inside of the flanges. While very light contact between the nipple and the flange works for some parents, increased friction usually results in pain and less milk. And so— if your nipples are rubbing and you feel uncomfortable, please try the next flange size up.*
  - ○ If there is a lot of room around your nipple in the flange tunnel, they are too large.

- Are your flanges centered?
  - ○ And off-center flange can cause your nipple to rub up against the inside of the tunnel. Reposition the flanges to see if this fixes the issue.

- Is your suction too high?
  - It is extremely rare to be pumping at the highest suction level.
  - The most common reason someone is pumping at the highest level is because their flanges are the wrong size, or their pump is not working correctly.
  - Too high a suction level can cause pain, and less milk to flow.
  - Turn your suction down, and then slowly go up to find your highest level of comfort.

- Does a lot of your breast seem to get pulled far into your flange no matter what you do?
  - Either your flange is too big, and/or you may have very stretchy areolar tissue, sometimes called "elastic nipples."
  - There are several flange cushions and inserts on the market to help with elastic nipple issues.
  - Finding as small a fit as possible without causing pain helps women with elastic nipples get comfortable.

- Is the base of your nipple getting sore?
  - Make sure you have a good flange fit.
  - Try applying coconut oil or nipple butter to your areolas, which will provide lubrication while you pump.
  - Try an insert that pads the flange.
  - Turn down your suction and work slowly up to an effective and comfortable level.

- How long are your pumping sessions?
  - A 15–minute double pumping session should be adequate to re-place a feeding if you have one baby. This is the equivalent of one 30–minute breastfeeding/chestfeeding session.
  - If you have twins, 25 minutes of double pumping should be ad-equate. This is the equivalent of 50 minutes of nursing.
  - Pumping for longer than these times tends to result in sore nip-ples, but not much more milk.

- o If you are trying to increase your supply, know that for many parents, more frequent sessions tend to work better than fewer, longer sessions and should help to decrease nipple pain.
  - I.e., three 15-minute pumping sessions over the course of a few hours are likely to yield significantly more milk than one 45-minute session.

- If nothing is working to resolve your pain, there might be a problem that is unrelated to pump logistics. Medical conditions such as thrush, vaso-spasms, nipple blisters, plugged ducts and mastitis are also a cause of breast and nipple pain. Call your health care provider and a lactation consultant to talk through these other possibilities.

REFERENCES

1. Parker LA, Sullivan S, Kruger C, Mueller M. Timing of milk expression following delivery in mothers delivering preterm very low birth weight infants: a randomized trial. *J Perinatol.* 2020; Aug;40(8):1236-1245. doi: 10.1038/s41372-020-0688-z.

2. Koroglu OA, Can N, Atikan BY, et al. Efficacy and maternal comfort of sequential versus simultaneous breast expression by mothers of critically ill newborns. *J Pediatr Res.* 2017; 4(4):211-215. doi: 10.4274/jpr.74436

3. Centers for Disease Control and Prevention. How to keep your breast pump kit clean: The essentials. Centers for Disease Control and Prevention website. Updated July 8, 2020. Accessed July 20, 2022. https://www.cdc.gov/healthywater/hygiene/healthychildcare/infantfeeding/breastpump.html

4. Zhang F, Yang Y, Bai T, et.al. Effect of pumping pressure on onset of lactation after caesarean section: A randomized controlled study. *Matern Child Nutr.* 2017; 14(1). doi: 10.1111/mcn.12486

5. Mayo Clinic Staff. Gestational diabetes. Mayo clinic website. Updated April 9, 2022. Accessed July 20, 2022. https://www.mayoclinic.org/diseases-conditions/gestational-diabetes/symptoms-causes/syc-20355339

6. Abramowski A, Ward R, Hamdan, AH. Neonatal Hypoglycemia. NIH National Library of Medicine website. Updated September 9, 2021. Accessed July 20, 2022. https://www.ncbi.nlm.nih.gov/books/NBK537105/

7. Juntereal N, Spatz D. Integrative review of antenatal milk expression and mother-infant outcomes during the first 2 weeks after birth. *J Obstet Gynecol Neonatal Nurs.* 2021; 50(6):659-668. doi: 10.1016/j.jogn.2021.07.003.

8. Centers for Disease Control and Prevention. Proper storage and preparation of breast milk. Centers for Disease Control and Prevention website. Updated January 24, 2022. Accessed July 20, 2022. https://www.cdc.gov/breastfeeding/recommendations/handling_breastmilk.htm

9. Eglash A, Simon L, and The Academy of Breastfeeding Medicine. ABM clinical protocol #8: Human milk storage information for home use for full-term infants, revised 2017. *Breastfeed Med.* 2017; 12(7):390-395. doi: 10.1089/bfm.2017.29047.aje

10. Qin Y, Shi W, Zhuang J, et al. Variations in melatonin levels in preterm and term human breast milk during the first month after delivery. *Sci Rep.* 2019; 9(1):17984. doi: 10.1038/s41598-019-54530-2

11. Teng ZW, Yang GQ, Wang LF, et al. Effects of the circadian rhythm on milk composition in dairy cows: Does day milk differ from night milk? *J Dairy Sci.* 2021; 104(7):8301-8313. doi: 10.3168/jds.2020-19679

12. American Academy of Pediatrics. Amount and schedule of baby formula feedings. Healthy Children website. Updated May 16, 2022. Accessed July 22, 2022. https://www.healthychildren.org/English/ages-stages/baby/formula-feeding/Pages/Amount-and-Schedule-of-Formula-Feedings.aspx

13. Kellams A, Harrel C, Omage S, Gregory C, Rosen-Carole C, and The Academy of Breastfeeding Medicine. ABM clinical protocol #3: Supplementary feedings in the healthy term breastfed neonate, re-

vised 2017. *Breastfeed Med.* 2017; 12(3):1-11. doi: 10.1089/bfm.2017.29038.aj

14. Foong SC, Tan ML, Foong WC, Marasco LA, Ho JJ, Ong JH. Oral galactagogues (natural therapies or drugs) for increasing breast milk production in mothers of non-hospitalized term infants. *Cochrane Database of Syst Rev.* 2020;(5): CD011505. doi: 10.1002/14651858.CD011505.pub2

15. von Wernsdorff M, Loef M, Tuschen-Caffier B, et al. Effects of open-label placebos in clinical trials: a systematic review and meta-analysis. *Sci Rep* 2021; 11(3855). doi: 10.1038/s41598-021-83148-6

16. Morton J. Maximizing milk production with hands-on pumping. Stanford Medicine. Accessed July 22, 2022. https://med.stanford.edu/newborns/professional-education/breastfeeding/maximizing-milk-production.html.

17. Walter MH, Abele H, Plappert CF. The role of oxytocin and the effect of stress during childbirth: Neurobiological basics and implications for mother and child. *Front. Endocrinol* 2021; Oct 27;12: 742236. doi: 10.3389/fendo.2021.742236

18. Centers for Disease Control and Prevention. Breastfeeding and special circumstances: Alcohol. Centers for Disease Control and Prevention website. Updated February 9, 2021. Accessed February 2, 2022. https://www.cdc.gov/breastfeeding/breastfeeding-special-circumstances/vaccinations-medications-drugs/alcohol.html

19. Shukri NH, Wells JC, Fewtrell M. The effectiveness of interventions using relaxation therapy to improve breastfeeding outcomes: A systematic review. *Maternal Child Nutr.* 2018 Apr; 14(2): e12563. doi: 10.1111/mcn.12563

20. Morton J. Hand expression of breastmilk. Stanford Medicine. Accessed February 2, 2022. https://med.stanford.edu/newborns/professional-education/breastfeeding/hand-expressing-milk.html

21. Rito AI, Buoncristiano M, Spinelli A, et al. Association between characteristics at birth, breastfeeding and obesity in 22 countries: The WHO European childhood obesity surveillance initiative–COSI 2015/2017. *Obes Facts.* 2019 12(2):226-243. doi: 10.1159/000500425

22. Bartok CJ, Ventura AK. Mechanisms underlying the association between breastfeeding and obesity. *Int J Pediatr Obes* 2009, 1-9

23. Li R, Magadia J, Fein SB, Grummer-Strawn LM. Risk of Bottle-feeding for Rapid Weight Gain During the First Year of Life. *Arch Pediatr Adolesc Med.* 2012;166(5):431–436. doi:10.1001/archpediatrics.2011.1665

24. Department of Labor. Frequently Asked Questions– Break Time for Nursing Mothers. Department of Labor website. Accessed on July 22, 2022. https://www.dol.gov/agencies/whd/nursing-mothers/faq

ABOUT THE AUTHOR:

Michelle McKeown Poole is a registered nurse (RN), international board certified lactation consultant (IBCLC) and holds a master's degree in counseling (MS). She has been helping parents through pregnancy, birth and newborn care for over 10 years, and loves every minute of it. Her techniques tear down old models of parenthood that produce anxiety, stress, guilt and fear, and create a new way of being that stresses comfort, confidence, ease and balance.

Visit bottleandboob.com to work with Michelle.

ABOUT THE ILLUSTRATOR:

Elizabeth McKeown holds a BFA in Fine Arts and Printmaking and loves creating art that makes you lean in a little closer. She figured out how to care for newborns by having three of her own and volunteered as a breastfeeding counselor for more than five years.

She effortlessly works whimsy and humor into her art, and is available to help you with your project: BebeKlim@gmail.com

ABOUT THE COVER DESIGN:

Monica Brown is a self-proclaimed "swiss army knife designer," specializing in motion graphics, print and presentation design. She loves working with small businesses and nonprofits. To learn more visit prettiegood.com.

Made in USA - Crawfordsville, IN
50223_9781734528718
11.02.2022 1345